MISSIONARY
MEDICINE©

A Guide for LDS Missionary Health

Senior Editor
Dr. Richard Justin Ingebretsen
Clinical Instructor of Medicine
University of Utah School of Medicine

ACKNOWLEDGMENT

We gratefully acknowledge Devon Hale, MD for reviewing the manuscript of this book

Research
Justin S. Coles
University of Utah School of Medicine
Salt Lake City, Utah

Graphics Design
Dillon W. Jensen
University of Utah School of Medicine
Salt Lake City, Utah

Proceeds from the sale of this book will be donated to The Church of Jesus Christ of Latter-day Saints' General Missionary Fund.

CONTRIBUTORS

Spencer Amundsen, MD
Department of Orthopaedic Surgery
Dartmouth Hitchcock Medical Center
Lebanon, New Hampshire
Brazil, Curitiba Mission

P. Egan Anderson
University of Utah School of Medicine
Salt Lake City, Utah
Germany, Frankfurt Mission

Scott Benson, MD
Department of Infectious Disease
University of Utah School of Medicine
Salt Lake City, Utah
Dominican Republic, Santa Domingo Mission

Justin S. Coles
University of Utah School of Medicine
Salt Lake City, Utah
Chile, Osorno Mission

Nelson Diamond
Medical Student, Duke University School of Medicine
Durham, North Carolina
Brazil, Maceio Mission

Donald B. Doty, MD
Adjunct Faculty, University of Utah School of Medicine
Salt Lake City, Utah
Vietnam Veteran

Gregory W. Ellis, MD
Psychiatry, Medical Director, The Center for Change
Salt Lake City, Utah
Japan, Tokyo South Mission

Paul Frandsen, MD
Adjunct Faculty, University of Utah School of Medicine
Emergency Department Intermountain Medical Center
Salt Lake City, Utah
Philippines, Cabanatuan Mission

Joseph C. Fyans, MD
Department of Physical Medicine and Rehabilitation
Jordan Valley Medical Center
Salt Lake City, Utah
Indiana, Indianapolis Mission

William Gochnour
University of Utah School of Medicine
Salt Lake City, Utah
Argentina, Resistencia Mission

Jonathan Guenter, MD
Adjunct Professor, Department of Surgery
University of Utah School of Medicine
Salt Lake City, Utah
Argentina, Buenos Aires South Mission

Harland N. Hayes, MD
Adjunct Faculty, University of Utah School of Medicine
Emergency Department Intermountain Medical Center
Salt Lake City, Utah
Tahiti, Papeete Mission

Nate Holman, MD
Department of Family Medicine
Ball Memorial Hospital
Muncie, Indiana
Germany, Frankfurt Mission

Richard J. Ingebretsen, MD, PhD
Clinical Instructor of Medicine
University of Utah School of Medicine
Salt Lake City, Utah
Washington DC Mission

Dillon W. Jensen
University of Utah School of Medicine
Salt Lake City, Utah
Norway, Oslo Mission

Adam Johnson, MD
Emergency Physician
St. John's Medical Center
Jackson, Wyoming
Stockholm, Sweden Mission

Benjamin Johnson, MD
Department of Anesthesia
University of Utah School of Medicine
Salt Lake City, Utah
Mexico City, North Mission

Eliza Johnson, MD
Department of Emergency Medicine
University of Utah School of Medicine
Salt Lake City, Utah
Hawaii, Honolulu Mission

Nate D. Kofford, MD, MSPH
Department of Anesthesia
Dartmouth Hitchcock Medical Center
Lebanon, New Hampshire
France, Bordeaux Mission

Jackson F. Lever, MD
Department of Ophthalmology
William Beaumont Hospital
Royal Oak, Michigan
Canada, Montreal Mission

Paul A. Schmutz, DDS
Dentistry, Wilderness Medicine
University of Utah School of Medicine
Salt Lake City, Utah
Pennsylvania, Pittsburgh Mission

Todd D. Sorensen
University of Utah School of Medicine
Salt Lake City, Utah
Honduras, Comayaguela Mission

Scott D. Williams, MD, MPH
Utah Department of Health, Past Executive Director
Division of Community and Family Health Services, Past
Director
Salt Lake City, Utah
Canada, Toronto Mission

Benjamin J. Wilson, MD
University of Utah School of Medicine
Salt Lake City, Utah
Alabama, Birmingham Mission

MEDICAL CARE ON YOUR MISSION

- Inform your mission president or designated health care coordinator of all medical issues, including any medications you are taking or any foods, medicines, or activities that you need to avoid.
- Report to your mission president if you experience any of the following:
  - Health problems beyond normal colds and other short term problems
  - Rapid pulse (100+ beats per minute at rest)
  - Fever of 101° F (38.3° C) for more than two days or any fever of 102° F (39° C) or above
  - Extreme weight loss or gain
  - Extreme thirst or urination
  - Persistent vomiting, headaches, dizziness, cough or rash
  - Swelling of the feet, legs, abdomen or face
  - Black-colored stools or bleeding during bowel movements
  - Diarrhea for more than two days
  - Serious injury
- This manual is designed to help you know when to call the mission president so that you can coordinate all medical care with him.
- Do not rely on members, friends, or family for diagnosing medical problems.
- Remember: Tuberculosis is a disease encountered by missionaries. It can be dormant (silent) for years. Therefore it is very important that you be checked for tuberculosis by your doctor when you return home from your mission.

TABLE OF CONTENTS

ABDOMINAL PAIN

Everyone experiences abdominal pain from time to time. Though most abdominal pain is short-lived and inconsequential, some causes of abdominal pain are true emergencies and require medical or surgical care. Missionaries may experience abdominal pain more frequently than they did prior to their missions because of changes in emotional stress, diet, and climate. Again, many cases of abdominal pain aren't emergencies, but if, after reading this chapter, you are concerned that your pain may be from a more serious cause, contact your mission doctor or seek medical attention immediately.

Below are some general guidelines. Without medical training, it can be difficult to determine the cause of abdominal pain. Though you may feel pain in one area of your abdomen, it may actually be caused by a problem in another area of your abdomen or body. For example, problems with the testicles or ovaries can also cause pain in the abdomen.

Causes of abdominal pain that will likely resolve without medical attention:

Note: There are many more causes of abdominal pain excluded from this list. Many causes of less serious abdominal pain share symptoms with serious causes of abdominal pain.

- Gas pain
- Constipation
- Heartburn / acid reflux
- Diarrhea with intestinal spasm
- Menstrual cramps

- Irritable bowel syndrome – irritation, gas, diarrhea, chronic abdominal discomfort
- Swollen lymph nodes in the abdomen – often after viral illnesses
- Ovarian cysts – often associated with the menstrual cycle and can cause sudden sharp pain or nagging pain for a few days
- Strained or pulled abdominal muscle – usually due to new exercise, or sudden twisting or jerking movements
- Gastroenteritis – vomiting and diarrhea from a virus or from food poisoning, usually lasting two days or less

Causes of abdominal pain that are more serious and require treatment:

- Appendicitis – inflammation or infection of the appendix (part of the large intestine), usually with pain on the lower right side of the abdomen, nausea, and decreased appetite
- Bladder or urinary tract infection – increased frequency of urination with burning and a sense of urgency during urination. Though generally not serious, if not treated it may progress to a serious kidney infection with fever, flank pain, and vomiting
- Kidney stone – sudden onset of intense flank pain that may come and go in waves and can also be associated with blood in your urine
- Endometriosis – causes pain in females during menstruation due to tissue from the uterus being abnormally located in the abdomen
- Inflammatory bowel disease – chronic fevers, generalized abdominal pain, and possible blood in your stools
- Intestinal blockage – abdominal bloating with nausea, vomiting, intense pain, and without bowel movements or passing of gas; most often occurs in those with previous abdominal surgeries
- Gallbladder infection – constant pain in the upper or right upper part of the abdomen, sometimes with fever, nausea, and vomiting

- Gallbladder stones – intense pain in the right upper part of the abdomen, often with eating, then resolving after minutes or hours; may lead to an infected gallbladder or pancreas inflammation
- Ovarian torsion – the ovary twists on itself, cutting off its blood supply, and causing very intense pain, often with nausea and vomiting
- Hernia – a bulge in the groin or scrotum
- Some parasite infections
- Testicular pain – may be caused by infection or swelling of the testicles, or twisting of a testicle may cut off its blood supply and cause intense pain
- Vaginal and pelvic infections

TREATMENT

Treat the cause of the abdominal pain. Get advice from the mission doctor.

WHEN TO SEE A DOCTOR

Seek help quickly if the pain is severe or associated with:

- Trauma, such as an accident or injury
- Pressure or pain in your chest
- Pain that is isolated to the right lower part or right upper part of your abdomen
- Duration of pain for more than 24 hours
- Loss of appetite for several hours
- Pain so severe that you can't sit still or need to curl into a ball to find relief
- Pain that is accompanied by bloody stools, persistent nausea and vomiting, skin that appears yellow, severe tenderness when you touch your abdomen, or swelling of the abdomen
- Swelling or pain of a testicle or the scrotum

- Persistent vomiting and or diarrhea with the inability to keep liquids down
- Vaginal bleeding that is excessive or pain that is significantly different from your normal menstrual cramps

ALLERGIES
(Allergic Reaction)

Missionaries find themselves in new environments with different pollens, foods, plants, and animals that may cause new allergies or make preexisting allergies worse. When you're allergic to something, your immune system mistakenly believes that this substance is harmful to your body. In an attempt to protect the body, the immune system reacts, causing symptoms of the allergic reaction. Every time you come into contact with that substance, you'll have an allergic reaction.

Allergic reactions can be mild, causing symptoms such as a runny nose, stuffy nose, or eye itching. A moderate allergic reaction may include "hives," or beefy, red, itchy patches of skin that can appear on different parts of the body. A severe, potentially life-threatening allergic reaction is called "anaphylaxis." Symptoms of anaphylaxis may include wheezing or difficulty breathing, hoarseness of the voice, swelling of the tongue, lips, or tissues in the throat, dizziness or loss of consciousness.

Common causes of allergic reactions include foods, medications, soaps, detergents, insect bites and stings, animals, plants, and some airborne particles. Sometimes a source or cause of the allergic reaction is never found.

TREATMENT

Medications are often used to treat allergies. Many effective medications are available to treat common allergies, and the mission doctor can help you to identify those that work for you. Antihistamines are the best ones. They might make you tired but are effective. If allowed, go to the local pharmacy and look for any antihistamines and follow the instructions. Common names are Dimetapp (Phenylephrine), Chlor-Trimeton (Pseudoephedrine), and Benadryl (Diphenhydramine). Some allergic reactions will require the use of prednisone, which is a steroid. Many rashes need steroids. You can rub steroids on as a cream or take it as a pill. Anaphylaxis might require a drug called epinephrine. If you are having trouble breathing, seek medical attention immediately.

Missionaries should avoid foods and other substances that are known to give them allergy symptoms. It's important to politely decline and explain your allergy when you are offered foods or are around pets to which you're allergic.

ANXIETY

Anxiety disorders continue to be the most common issues that missionaries struggle with during their mission. Fortunately anxiety disorders are usually quite treatable. A significant part of that treatment is early recognition and treatment of the anxiety. What follows is a brief description of some of the most common conditions.

In general, anxiety is a feeling of worry, fear, nervousness, or stress. Anxiety is a normal response to a new or different situation. Anxiety helps as we adapt to a new event in a way that maximizes our success and safety in that new situation. Anxiety helps us to learn and readjust with success and safety through periods of our lives. Everyone will experience this emotion.

Missionaries will experience anxiety while on their missions and most will overcome the feelings. However, for some, anxiety becomes the master. It ceases to be productive, but instead is destructive. This often occurs to missionaries who have previously had bad experiences with anxiety. Anxiety, which was once helpful, now becomes so intense that it becomes a big problem. When anxiety is this strong, it tends to preoccupy or distract us.

Depression can cause anxiety. Overwhelming feelings of anxiety can occur as you become aware of how the depression is stripping you of your ability to successfully perform your daily tasks. Furthermore, some kinds of depression are ravaged by continual intense feelings of anxiety. These kinds of depression are termed "anxious depressions." Anxious depressions are common. A red flag should go up when this type of depression is occurring. This is because the extreme levels of anxiety accompanying this kind of depression are difficult to bear.

Anxiety can be a self-reinforcing event. The desire to relieve anxiety can itself become a source of stress, often worsening the emotional burden. Simply talking through the anxiety with your mission president or writing to your family can often make a big difference. However, attempting to deal with these problems alone sometimes leads to destructive decisions, including even self-harming behaviors. It is of the utmost importance that this situation be recognized and professionally treated. As with most psychological conditions, recognizing anxiety early can help you avoid more difficult problems later. So watch for such behaviors both in yourself and your companion.

Adjusting to a change can generate emotions of anxiety. Such changes include learning a new language, transferring to a new area, leaving home, working with a new companion or coping with a disappointment. Such events may provoke intense anxiety or depression. This is called an adjustment disorder.

TREATMENT

The key to reducing the intensity of your anxiety and depression lies in changing your perspective. It is all about changing your expectations and regaining access to positive support and routines.. Other effective methods include talking and writing letters or emails to trusted leaders, friends or family. Reviewing written material that has been approved by your mission president can help as well. Refocusing your efforts in this direction can help you regain your confidence.

Remember, anxiety is a normal part of your life and of your missionary experience. Without anxiety we would miss many of life's important learning opportunities. Feelings of anxiety do not signal a need to depart from your missionary service, but they do prompt you to act.

The Church has anticipated that you will have many new and different experiences during your mission. Church leaders are mindful of you and have generated resources to assist you in overcoming your anxiety as you strive to fulfill your mission. The principles of obedience to mission rules and reading the mission handbook and written materials (such as *Preach My Gospel*) will help you overcome anxiety during your mission service.

Simple routines related to personal study, healthy diet and regular correspondence with your family and church leaders will strengthen your emotional and physical health. They will also help you discover and build up your spiritual strength.

BACK PAIN

A lot of missionaries get back pain. To help treat back pain it is useful to know about the back. It is a complex structure made up of 33 vertebrae, over 30 muscles, numerous ligaments, multiple joints, and inter-vertebral discs. So when talking about back pain there are many things that can cause it. Some common things that missionaries do to cause back pain are:

- Wearing backpacks (overloaded or improperly worn)
- Riding bikes
- Sleeping in an odd position
- Improper lifting of heavy objects

Whatever the cause might be, the injuries that can be sustained, causing back pain can range from very mild to very severe. Sometimes the pain is hard to accurately diagnose without proper medical attention and examinations. Causes of back pain include:

- Muscle strains and sprains
- Herniated discs

The most common cause of back pain is due to muscle sprains and strains. This happens when a force, twist, or pull is applied to one or several of the muscles or ligaments in the back. As a result, they are stretched way too far causing pain in these specific muscles or ligaments. Back pain can also be accompanied by referred pain. This means that pain can travel down the legs. If you feel pain going down your leg, there is probably something wrong with the discs in your back and will likely need more care.

TREATMENT

Medications to manage pain can be helpful to alleviate symptoms. Ibuprofen will help relieve the pain and reduce the swelling of the muscles.

Back pain that is caused by herniated disks requires professional medical attention. Herniated disks can also cause referred pain and sensations in the leg. See a doctor if there is prolonged back pain that is not improving.

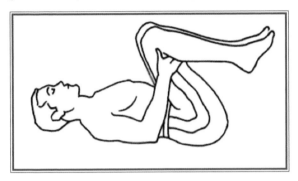

One exercise that is useful is to lie on your back, put your hands behind the knees and slowly pull your knees up to your chest. Hold them there for a second or two and then slowly release your legs. Continue doing this for about 5 minutes and then relax. Repeat this exercise every hour as possible. This will help to stretch your muscles and open the vertebrae up, relieving back pain.

PREVENTION

The best prevention for some of these back injuries is to simply use items correctly.

- Bike seats should be high enough so that your leg is straight. Be sure that it is not too high so that your knee locks when reaching the pedal at its lowest point.

- Backpacks should be worn so that the weight is distributed evenly over your back. The best way to check if a backpack is being worn properly is to lengthen or shorten the straps so that the bottom of the bag reaches about the small of your back. Also, avoid overloading a backpack as this increases the risk of injury.
- Shoulder bags should have light loads and should be alternated between shoulders so as to not strain back muscles.
- To avoid back pain from sleeping, sleep with a pillow between your knees, as this helps to reduce strain and pressure on the spine and also give it better support.
- Avoid exercises that put pressure on your back or cause your back to hurt such as weight lifting and squatting with weights.

BITES AND STINGS

Missionaries are going to see a lot of dogs and cats on their mission. If you are bitten by a dog or a cat, here are some general guidelines for care:

- Wounds that do not break the skin can be treated with ice and anti-inflammatory medications such as ibuprofen.
- For wounds that do break the skin:
  - Direct pressure should be applied to the bite to stop the bleeding if needed.
  - The wound should be flushed with clean soapy water as soon as possible.
  - The cleaner the water the better.
  - Dress the wound with bandages.
- If the wound involves a joint (especially on the hand) it is an emergency and you should see a doctor as soon as possible.
- Cat bites are more likely to become infected than dog bites, so make sure to get treated with antibiotics.
- Call the mission doctor if you have been bitten by a cat or a dog.
- Rabies is a concern. Find the dog and check for rabies for 10 days. If you can't find the dog, contact the missionary doctor to make decisions about obtaining the rabies vaccine.

Prevention

- Do not kiss a dog.
- Do not lean over and pet a dog on the head.
- Do not physically separate fighting dogs.

- Never take a bone or toy away from an unfamiliar dog.
- Do not approach a nursing dog.

MOSQUITOES

Mosquitoes transmit disease that will cause the deaths of 1 in 17 people alive today. Worldwide, 300-500 million people contract malaria annually. Of those, 3 million will die. Other mosquito-borne illnesses include encephalitis, yellow fever, dengue fever, and other diseases. Mosquito-borne diseases found in the United States are eastern equine encephalitis, western equine encephalitis, St. Louis encephalitis, La Crosse encephalitis, and West Nile Virus. Mosquitoes are attracted by warm skin, and moisture. They are also attracted to the smell of soap, detergents, and perfume.

Prevention

- If you are serving in an area that has malaria, be sure to avoid bites and take the medicine that the Church has recommended.
- Malaria mosquitoes are most active at dusk, so staying indoors during that time will decrease the likelihood of being bitten.
- Dengue Fever mosquitos bite during the day.
- Using mosquito netting around your bed can help reduce the chances of getting bitten during the night. If you don't put a net over your bed, you can put a net over your window.
- Wear clothing that covers as much skin as possible such as long sleeves and long socks.
- Wear clothing that is tightly woven, such as nylon, and is loose fitting so that a mosquito cannot bite through the clothing.
- Wear insect repellent on uncovered skin.
- DEET is the gold standard for insect repellents.
  - It is sold in formulations of 5% to 35%.
  - Use formulations of 30% to 35% in malaria areas.

- ▪ Do not use sunscreens that contain DEET, as sunscreens need to be used liberally and often, whereas DEET should be used less often.
- Apply permethrin to clothing and bedding, especially mosquito netting
- Permethrin is a naturally occurring compound with insecticidal and repellent properties that will remain on clothing for weeks when properly applied.
- See the appendix on permethrin for more information.

SPIDERS

Many spiders are venomous, but only a few are dangerous to humans. Many spiders do not have enough venom to affect a human, and many spiders do not have fangs large enough to penetrate human skin. Dangerous North American spiders include the black widow, brown recluse and hobo spiders. Some countries such as New Zealand do not have poisonous spiders, while other countries such as Australia have a number of deadly spiders.

Treatment

- Catch the spider, if possible, to allow for identification.
- Cleanse the bite with soap and water.
- For pain relief, use a cold compress or ice pack and medications like acetaminophen (Tylenol) / paracetamol or ibuprofen.
- Many spider bites will cause a small allergic reaction. See the chapter on allergic reactions for treatment.
- Get medical attention if you become sick.

TICKS

Ticks transmit many serious diseases such as Lyme disease, Rocky Mountain spotted fever, Colorado tick fever, and Tularemia. They are found in areas replete with weeds, shrubs, and trails. They will often be found at forest boundaries where deer and other mammals reside. They will sit on low hanging shrubs with their legs outstretched until an animal or a person passes. Refer to chapter on ticks for more information.

Prevention

- Check clothing and exposed skin for ticks.
- Tuck shirts into pants and pants into socks.
- Wear smooth, tightly woven, loose fitting clothing.
- Soak or spray clothing with permethrin.
- Wear DEET insect repellent.

Treatment

- Use tweezers or the tips of your fingers to grasp the tick as close to the skin surface as possible.
- Pull the tick straight upward with steady even pressure to remove it.
- Wash the bite with soap and water, and then wash your hands after the tick has been removed.

The 'DO NOTS' of tick removal:

- Do not use petroleum jelly.
- Do not use fingernail polish.
- Do not use rubbing alcohol.
- Do not use a hot match.
- Do not use gasoline.
- Do not twist or jerk the tick, as this will most likely cause incomplete removal of the tick. Ticks do not have heads but do have a small sucking probe.

SCORPIONS

Scorpions don't bite, they sting. They are often found lurking in shoes or on clothes. So if you are serving in an area where scorpions are found, make sure you look before you put on your clothes. If you are stung by a scorpion, the main effect will be pain at the site of the sting. Ice is very useful for a scorpion sting as it helps to neutralize the venom. You can take acetaminophen (Tylenol) / paracetamol or ibuprofen for pain relief as well.

BEES, WASPS, HORNETS, ANTS

The bite from an ant, wasp, hornet or a bee will almost always cause a small irritating bite and often a small local allergic reaction (see the chapter on allergic reactions). But the most serious problem is the possibility of having a serious allergic reaction called anaphylaxis.

- A local reaction is the most common reaction. It consists of a small red patch that burns and itches.
- The generalized reaction (anaphylaxis) consists of diffuse red skin, hives, swelling of lips and tongue, wheezing, abdominal cramps and diarrhea.
- Stings to the mouth and throat are more serious, as they may cause airway swelling.

Prevention/Treatment

- Bees and wasps are attracted to rotten fruit and fruit syrups.
- Frequent cleaning of garbage areas and proper disposal of old fruit will decrease bee and wasp attraction.
- Scrape away the stinger in a horizontal fashion using a card.
- Wash the site with soap and water.
- Place a cold compress or ice pack on the site.
- Take acetaminophen (Tylenol) / paracetamol or ibuprofen for pain relief.
- Topical steroid creams (hydrocortisone cream) and antihistamines (Benadryl) can help decrease swelling.
- If hives occur with wheezing and respiratory difficulty, then epinephrine (Epi-Pen) should be given immediately.

- Pepcid or Zantac should be used early in treatment.
- An epinephrine injection can be repeated 5 to 10 minutes after the initial injection.
- Prednisone (a steroid) and an antihistamine should also be taken, especially in situations when epinephrine is used.
- Prednisone and antihistamines can be used to help treat the rash
- The above medications should only be given under the direction of a physician.
- You should call 911 or go directly to the hospital for any sign of the systemic reaction called anaphylaxis (breathing trouble, rash, headache, lightheadedness).

BLISTERS

A blister is a small pocket of fluid within the upper layers of the skin. Most blisters are filled with a clear fluid called serum or plasma. This fluid cushions the tissue underneath, protecting it from further damage and allowing it to heal.

However, blisters can be filled with blood (known as blood blisters) or with pus (if they become infected).

A blister may form when the skin has been damaged by friction, heat, sunburn, cold exposure, or chemical exposure. If friction continues without intervention, blisters enlarge and rupture, leading to painfully exposed deeper layers of skin.

TREATMENT

- If a small blister or hot spot forms, use Blist-o-ban or equivalent to protect the area. This is the most effective way to protect a blister. Another way to protect a blister is done by cutting a hole the size of the blister in a piece of moleskin or medical tape. Then secure the moleskin or medical tape over the blister to act as a shield to the area. Anchor the moleskin with benzoin or a similar adhesive product if available, and secure with tape. Build up several layers as necessary.

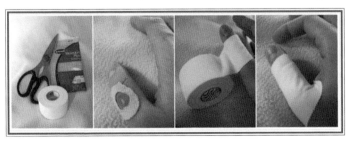

- Do not open or puncture small blisters. The unbroken skin over a blister provides a natural barrier to infection. Ideally, blisters should be allowed to break on their own after the skin underneath has healed.
- If the blister is large (quarter-sized) or ruptured, wash the area and puncture the base of the blister with a sterile needle or safety pin. Remove the external flap of skin from the blister, apply an antibiotic ointment, and cover the blister with a sterile dressing. This can be protected with moleskin, mole foam or medical tape.
- Inspect the area daily for signs of infection (increasing pain, redness, or draining pus). If an intact blister becomes infected, drain it, cut away the dead skin, and then seek medical attention.

PREVENTION

- Blisters on the feet can be prevented by wearing comfortable, well-fitting shoes and clean socks.
- Blisters are more likely to develop on skin that is moist, so changing socks frequently or wearing socks that wick away moisture will aid those with particularly sweaty feet.
- Before going for long walks, it is also important to ensure that your shoes have been properly broken in.
- Even before a "hot" or irritated area on the foot is felt, taping a protective layer of padding or taping a friction-reducing material (like Blist-o-ban, athletic tape, or duct tape) between the affected area and the footwear can prevent the formation of a blister.
- Use sunscreen to prevent sunburn blisters – or better still, cover your skin with clothes.

BOILS
(Large Painful Pimples)

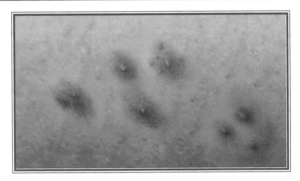

If you have a large painful lump on your skin, you might have a boil. This is a skin infection and looks like a very large pimple. Boils usually get worse quickly and will become softer, larger and more painful over several days. Often a pocket of pus will develop just under the skin. The most common places for boils to appear are on the face, neck, armpits, shoulders and buttocks. When a boil forms on an eyelid it is called a sty. When it forms at the base of the spine it is called a pilonidal cyst.

CAUSES

Boils are usually caused by bacteria called *Staphylococcus* (staph). This germ can be present on normal skin. It enters the body through tiny breaks in the skin or by traveling down a hair to the follicle. However, certain health problems make people more susceptible to skin infections such as boils. For example, diabetes, poor nutrition and poor cleanliness may increase the risk of getting boils. The staph bacteria are found in the nose, so if you touch or pick your nose and then touch your skin, you might cause boils.

WHEN TO SEEK MEDICAL CARE

Boils usually do not require immediate medical attention. But, there are certain times that you should seek medical care more quickly:

- If you have a boil and start running a fever.
- The skin around the boil turns red or red streaks appear.
- The pain becomes severe.
- The boil does not drain.
- A second boil appears.

TREATMENT

You can try to treat boils yourself – but only smaller boils. If your boil is bigger than a dime or if it has a lot of redness around it, seek medical attention rather than trying to deal with it yourself. To treat a small boil yourself:

- Soak the boil in warm water. This will decrease the pain and help draw the pus to the surface. (You can make a warm compress by soaking a wash cloth in warm water and squeezing out the excess moisture.)
- Once the boil comes to a head, it will burst. This usually occurs within several days of its appearance.
- When the boil starts draining, wash it with soap until the pus is gone.
- Apply an antibiotic ointment.

PREVENTION

Help prevent boils by washing your clothes, sheets and towels, and by treating minor cuts and scrapes. Don't pick or touch your nose. The bacteria that causes boils "lives" in your nose. Shower and wash your hands regularly.

PILONIDAL CYST

If a boil occurs at the base of the spine near the crack in your buttocks, you probably have a pilonidal cyst. This is a special type of a boil and always needs medical attention.

BURNS

If you are burned, run cool water or place a cool, damp cloth over the affected area. That will help relieve the pain. What you do next is determined by how deep the burn is and how large an area it covers on your skin.

Superficial Burns

The skin is reddened and painful, but without blistering. A common example of a superficial burn is a sunburn. While painful, this is the easiest type of burn to treat.

Partial Thickness Burns

The skin is blistered, and deeper layers of the skin are exposed and red.

Full Thickness Burns

All layers of the skin have been burned. The flesh may be charred, but the victim feels no pain from a full-thickness burn because the nerve endings are destroyed. Partial thickness burns may surround the full-thickness burn. Full-thickness burns require immediate medical attention.

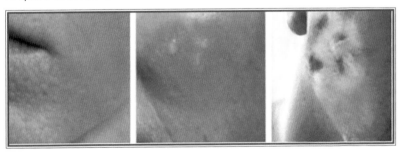

Superficial   Partial Thickness   Full Thickness

TREATMENT

For Superficial Burns

Treat superficial burns with aloe vera gel. For comfort, cool the area with a damp cloth. Use ibuprofen or acetaminophen (Tylenol) / paracetamol for pain.

For Partial and Full Thickness Burns

Call the mission doctor and seek medical attention. If you need to treat the wound yourself until you can get help, here are some guidelines:

- Gently clean the burn with cool water to remove loose skin and debris.
- Trim away all loose skin with scissors.
- Blisters larger than the size of a nickel should be drained, and the skin trimmed away.
- Apply a thin layer of antibacterial ointment to the burn and cover it with a non-sticking, clean dressing. Change the dressing at least once a day.
- If you have placed ice on the wound, do not ice it for more than 15 minutes as more damage may occur.
- Use pain medicines such as ibuprofen to help manage the pain.

When to Take a Burn Victim to the Hospital

Go to the hospital or a medical facility immediately in any of the following conditions:

- If the victim has a full-thickness burn
- If the burn involves the face, hands, feet, or genitals
- If the burn is an electrical burn
- If the burn is complicated by smoke inhalation
- If the burn victim is medically ill

CANKER SORES
(Sores inside the Mouth)

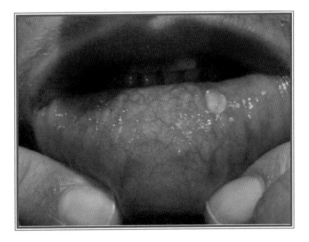

Most missionaries have had or will get a canker sore. People can get these painful sores on the tongue or on the inside of the cheeks and lips. The good news is that canker sores are not contagious like some other mouth sores, such as cold sores.

The exact cause of most canker sores is unknown. Certain foods – including citrus or acidic fruits and vegetables (such as lemons, oranges, pineapples, apples, figs, tomatoes, and strawberries) – can trigger a canker sore or make the problem worse. Sometimes a sharp tooth surface or dental appliance, such as braces, might also trigger canker sores. There may be a connection between canker sores and stress.

TREATMENT

There is no known treatment that is truly effective. However, canker sores generally will resolve on their own. Some people have success gargling salt water. Take one tablespoon of salt and dissolve it in a glass of warm water. Gargle and swish the salt water in your mouth, and then spit it out. Various over-the-counter medicines (like carbamide peroxide) can help to take the sting out of canker sores. Certain prescription medications may need to be taken if you have canker sores more than three times per year or they are severe enough that you aren't able to eat.

Watch what you eat when you have a canker sore. Spicy foods and acidic foods such as lemons or tomatoes can be extremely painful on these open wounds. Anything sharp, such as nuts or potato chips, can poke or rub the sore and can also cause pain. Be careful when you brush your teeth, too. It's important to keep your mouth clean, but brushing the sore itself with a toothbrush can make it worse. If you have canker sores that do not get better after a few weeks, if the sores keep coming back, if they make you feel so sick that you don't want to eat, or if you have a high fever with your sores, see the mission doctor.

COLD SORES
(Sores on the Lips)

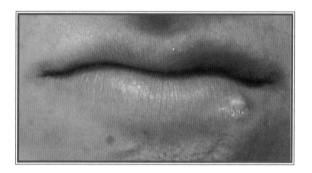

Cold sores are small and somewhat painful blisters caused by the herpes simplex virus (HSV). Cold sores usually show up on or around a person's lips, but they can also sometimes be inside the mouth, on the face, or even on or inside the nose. While these places are the most common, cold sores can appear anywhere on the body.

A person who has HSV doesn't always have sores. The virus can stay dormant in the body and then periodically become activated, causing cold sores. Not everyone who gets the herpes simplex virus develops cold sores, though. In some people, the virus stays asleep permanently.

Cold sores can be brought on by infections, fever, stress, sunlight, cold weather, hormone changes in menstruation or pregnancy, tooth extractions, and certain foods and drugs. In a lot of people, the cause is unpredictable.

HOW IT IS SPREAD

Cold sores are contagious. If you have a cold sore, people around you can easily be infected with HSV. The virus spreads through direct contact – through touching affected skin – but can still be passed on even if a sore is not yet visible. HSV can also be spread by sharing a cup, eating utensils, lip balm, or lipstick with someone who is infected.

Herpes simplex virus also can spread if a person touches the cold sore and then touches his or her mouth, nose, eyes, or an area of the skin with a cut on it. So it's best not to mess with a cold sore – don't pick, pinch, or squeeze it.

TREATMENT

Cold sores normally go away on their own within 7 to 10 days. And although no medications can make the infection go away, prescription drugs and creams are available that can shorten the length of the outbreak and make the cold sore less painful. If you have a cold sore, it's important to see a doctor if:

- You have another health condition that has weakened your immune system
- The sores don't heal by themselves within 7 to 10 days
- You get cold sores frequently
- You have signs of a bacterial infection, such as fever, pus, or spreading redness

To make yourself more comfortable when you have cold sores, you can apply ice or anything cool to the area. You also can take an over-the-counter pain reliever, such as acetaminophen / paracetamol or ibuprofen.

COLDS

DESCRIPTION

The common cold often causes runny nose, nasal congestion, sore throat, cough, and just plain feeling sick. Since it is a viral infection, antibiotics are not effective against the common cold. Symptoms from most common colds resolve in 7-10 days.

Sore throat is sometimes a symptom of a more serious condition distinct from the common cold, such as strep throat, which may require medical diagnosis and treatment with appropriate antibiotics. A sore throat without a runny nose or cough that lasts for more than a few days is more likely to be from a bacterial infection. If you have these symptoms, you should be checked by a doctor for a bacterial infection, which may require antibiotics.

HOW IT IS SPREAD

The common cold spreads very easily and rapidly. The viruses multiply mainly in the nose, so there are large quantities of viruses in the nasal fluid of people with colds. The highest concentration of cold virus in mucous occurs during the first three days of infection. This is when infected persons are most contagious.

Cold viruses are present in the droplets of coughs and sneezes. Cold viruses contaminate the hands of infected people as a result of nose blowing, covering sneezes, and touching the nose. Also, cold viruses may contaminate objects and surfaces in the area of a cold sufferer. Young children are the major carriers of cold viruses and are a particularly good source of virus-containing nasal secretions.

Experiments have demonstrated that a cold virus readily transfers from the skin and hands of a cold sufferer to the hands and fingers of another person during periods of brief contact. Also, cold viruses readily transfer to the hands as a result of touching contaminated objects and surfaces.

TREATMENT

Over-the-counter products may help to reduce the symptoms associated with the common cold and sore throats, but they do not speed recovery. Pain relievers such as aspirin, ibuprofen, and acetaminophen (Tylenol) / paracetamol can reduce pain due to sore throats and headaches. Products containing local anesthetics such as benzocaine (Cepacol Maximum) provide temporary relief from sore throat pain. Topical nasal decongestants such as Afrin and Neo-Synephrine may provide relief from nasal congestion, but they should only be used for a few days. The oral medicine, Sudafed may help relieve nasal congestion, while antihistamines such as Benadryl and Chlor-Trimeton might help dry excess mucous and reduce sneezing. The cough suppressant dextromethorphan may be recommended at bedtime to facilitate sleep.

PREVENTION

- Wash your hands or use hand sanitizer often.
- Avoid touching your eyes, nose and mouth. If you blow your nose, wash your hands before touching your mouth or eyes.
- Limit contact with people who are sick. If you don't want a cold, you probably don't want to intentionally expose yourself to people who have a cold. If you must, wash your hands afterwards.
- Eat healthy.
- Rest is important. Getting the full 8 hours of sleep as directed by the missionary handbook and keeping as close to your normal routine as possible is very effective.
- Drink water and stay warm and dry.

DENGUE FEVER

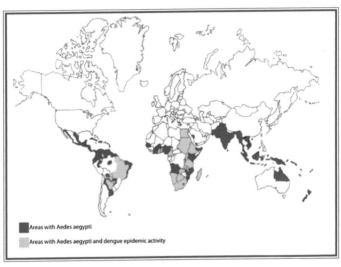

Areas with Aedes aegypti

Areas with Aedes aegypti and dengue epidemic activity

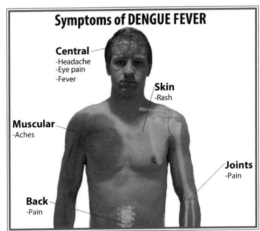

Symptoms of DENGUE FEVER

Central
-Headache
-Eye pain
-Fever

Skin
-Rash

Muscular
-Aches

Joints
-Pain

Back
-Pain

Missionaries will serve in areas around the world where diseases are found that are not common in the United States.

One of these diseases is called dengue fever. You should be aware of the symptoms and how to prevent it.

Dengue fever (pronounced DENG-gay) is a disease caused by a family of viruses that are carried by mosquitoes – usually the Aedes aegypti mosquito. It is an illness with the sudden onset of headache, fever, exhaustion, severe joint and muscle pain, swollen glands, and a rash. The presence of three symptoms – fever, rash, and pain (headache or other pains) – is particularly characteristic of dengue. Most people will recover on their own but it is debilitating.

Dengue is common throughout the tropics and subtropics. Outbreaks have occurred in the Caribbean, including Puerto Rico, the U.S. Virgin Islands, Cuba, and Central America. Cases have also been found in Tahiti, the South Pacific, Southeast Asia, the West Indies, India, and the Middle East.

HOW IT IS SPREAD

Dengue is transmitted through mosquito bites.

TREATMENT

If you suspect that you have dengue fever, call the mission doctor. The diagnosis of dengue fever is usually made based on your symptoms rather than a blood test. Because dengue is caused by a virus, there is no specific medicine or antibiotic to treat it. For typical dengue fever, the treatment is mainly for the relief of the symptoms while the disease runs its course. Resting and drinking plenty of fluids can help with recovery. However, if you start to bleed from your nose, gums or have bruising in your skin, you might have a more severe form of Dengue Fever called Dengue Hemorrhagic Fever and you will need medical professional care.

PREVENTION

To prevent dengue fever (and other mosquito-borne diseases) avoid being bitten by mosquitoes that usually bite during the day. In mosquito-infested areas you should always use personal protection such as long sleeve shirts and mosquito repellant sprays that contain DEET. Trim long grass and keep foliage to a minimum, especially in times of rain. Remove all objects from your yard that could possibly contain standing water.

DEPRESSION

The purpose of this chapter is to help you understand depression and to assist you in completing the missionary work that you set out to perform. Fortunately, not every missionary will suffer from depression. The Church, its leaders, and your mission president have prepared and put into place many resources designed to reduce the likelihood that you will ever experience this illness.

What follows are simple working descriptions of some common forms of depression. Knowing about the types of depression will help you to identify and resolve them more quickly while serving your mission.

It is important for you to involve your mission president early on and then every step of the way as you overcome depression. It is also important that you communicate with your companion, mission leaders, and your family.

Depression is a very common medical condition. Many, many millions of people currently suffer from depression, including missionaries. Missionaries with depression often lose their ability to manage their daily missionary activities. So how do you recognize and treat depression? Understanding what depression looks and feels like are the first steps in its successful treatment. Hesitating and denying the presence of the symptoms of depression may permit it to grow worse. Much like any health condition—prevention and treatment are the keys to staying in the best of health.

WHAT IS DEPRESSION?

The most common depression is called classic depression. In fact, it is often referred to simply as "depression." It is more than mere sadness. It requires that on a daily basis for at least two weeks you have had at least five of the nine symptoms listed below:

- An unusually sad mood
- A reduced ability to experience pleasure or interest in your day-to-day activities
- A change in your appetite that often causes a change in your weight
- Having significant trouble with sleeping
- Persisting fatigue or loss of your physical energy
- A change in the pace of your speech and/or physical movements
- Feelings of worthlessness or excessive guilt
- A reduced ability to think and concentrate
- Having recurring thoughts about death

If you have 5 out of 9 of these symptoms, you probably have depression. Talk with your mission president. He might refer you to a person trained in treating depression. They might start you on several different successful therapies. Fortunately, depression for the most part is responsive to treatment. Some of the treatment plans include:

- Changes in your diet and sleep habits
- Talk therapy
- Light therapy to kick-start your brain into making more natural "feel good" chemicals
- Medicine such as vitamin D or other minerals, as well as antidepressant and anti-anxiety medications

Some forms of depression can go undetected or misunderstood because of the uniqueness of their presentation. Just remember, they all have the same basic symptoms that have been described above. What follows are a few details concerning specific types of depression.

ADJUSTMENT REACTION (HOMESICKNESS)

This means a missionary is having difficulty adjusting to a new situation. Homesickness is a common type of adjustment reaction depression. It is particularly stressful for a missionary. Being away from your home, friends, and family puts into motion the symptoms of depression. If the situation goes away, or if you learn to adapt to the changes it presents, the depressive symptoms go away as well. One friend in this situation is time. As time goes on, you learn to make new friends and develop a new support system, and you will make a new home. The feelings of depression will then subside. Write letters or send emails home to get support from family and friends. Communicate frequently with your mission president and mission leaders to get their perspective, as they have been through it before. Live your mission one month at time – so to speak – until the symptoms have subsided. Change is the key here, even if it takes a few weeks or months.

Sometimes you are unable to change the situation – like dealing with a difficult transfer or companionship. This is another type of adjustment reaction. If you choose to focus on all that you cannot change, you may begin to foster feelings of helplessness and hopelessness.

On the other hand, if you focus on what you can change, you can improve your situation and your symptoms will go away. For example, you can improve your interpersonal communication skills. As you make this change, your situation will improve as you learn to communicate better with your companion. This process will help you to regain your sense of control and reduce your stress.

Learning how to regain your sense of internal control over external events that you thought were out of your control is the key to overcoming the symptoms of depression caused by an adjustment reaction.

Learning such positive and effective coping skills may require some effort on your part. You can draw from experiences that you had before your mission. Keeping open communication with supportive family, companions and your mission president can add to this process. At times, reading and careful study will assist you in learning how others have accomplished this change of perspective.

Should these efforts prove inadequate in moving you forward in your work to adapt to the situation, your mission president might have you talk with a counselor who can assist you in this process.

ATYPICAL DEPRESSION

The key feature of an atypical depression is a symptom known as "mood reactivity." Simply put, "mood reactivity" means that your depressed mood temporarily lifts when you have something good happen or anticipate something positive will happen (e.g., being around missionary friends or having something that you have hoped and worked for turn out). In classic depression, your mood stays depressed even when things around you are pleasant and going right.

Some of the expected depressive symptoms are backwards:

- Instead of being unable to sleep, you want to sleep all of the time.
- Rather than losing your appetite, you want to eat everything in sight — and you gain the weight to prove it.

Others are intensified:

- More than simply moving or speaking slowly, you feel as though your arms and legs are carrying heavy weights — like walking through a swimming pool
- More than simple feelings of guilt or hopelessness, you begin to have the sense that others are persistently rejecting or criticizing you.

SEASONAL DEPRESSION

Seasonal depression refers to a depression that comes on at the same time or season of the year. This often happens during the winter months if you're serving in a place where there is decreased daylight during the winter season.

The treatment of seasonal depression can involve the use of special lights. The lights mimic normal morning sunlight (without damaging your eyes). You awake one hour before the day's scheduled sunrise and peer into the light. Over the subsequent week your brain is tricked into thinking that it is spring or summer.

The result of this trick is a remission of your depression. It occurs because your brain is prompted (by the light therapy) to resume making normal amounts of materials that build, store and transport your natural "feel-good chemicals." You should continue on the light therapy until the season draws to its natural close.

CONCLUSION

Depression is common. It has many forms, some of which are discussed above. These details are for your use in discerning how best to recognize and treat your depression.

Use this knowledge to prevent and treat depression and to move forward in protecting your emotional health. This information is meant to supplement the countless resources already put into place by the Church for your benefit. Many of those resources are built into the mission rules and guidelines.

The Church and its leaders are well aware that your mission may be potentially stressful at times. They are likewise sensitive to the fact that you may experience disappointment and despair during your mission service. For this purpose they have and will continue to provide you with resources to accomplish the mission on which you have embarked.

DIARRHEA

Diarrhea is a common problem in developing countries where water is frequently contaminated. In most cases the loose, watery stools and abdominal cramps that characterize diarrhea last only a couple of days. Missionaries in some parts of the world are very prone to have diarrhea several times while serving.

Diarrhea may cause a loss of significant amounts of water and salts. Most cases of diarrhea resolve on their own without treatment. Bacterial or parasitic infections sometimes cause bloody stools, and fever may accompany these infections as well.

See a doctor if:

- Your diarrhea (watery stools) persists beyond three days.
- You become dehydrated — as evidenced by excessive thirst, dry mouth or skin, little or no urination, severe weakness, dizziness or lightheadedness, or dark-colored urine.
- You have severe abdominal or rectal pain.
- You have bloody or black stools.
- You have a temperature of more than 102°F (39°C).

CAUSES

The most common causes of diarrhea include:

- **Viruses.** Viral diarrhea spreads easily but usually resolves without treatment.

- **Bacteria and parasites.** Contaminated food or water can transmit bacteria and parasites to your body. Diarrhea caused by bacteria and parasites can be common when traveling in developing countries and is often called traveler's diarrhea.
- **Medications.** Many medications can cause diarrhea, most commonly antibiotics. Antibiotics can destroy both good and bad bacteria, which can disturb the natural balance of bacteria in your intestines.

Other causes

- **Lactose.** A sugar found in milk and milk products, lactose is a common cause of diarrhea in some people.
- **Artificial sweeteners.** Sorbitol and mannitol, artificial sweeteners found in chewing gum and other sugar-free products, can cause diarrhea in some otherwise healthy people.
- **Other digestive disorders.** Chronic diarrhea (lasting more than four weeks) has a number of other causes, such as Crohn's disease, ulcerative colitis, celiac disease, and irritable bowel syndrome.

TREATMENT

Drinking fluids is very important during bouts of diarrhea to prevent dehydration, which is the loss of vital fluids and electrolytes (sodium and potassium).

Although water is extremely important in preventing dehydration, it does not contain electrolytes. Good choices to help maintain electrolyte levels include broth or soups (which contain sodium) and fruit juices, soft fruits, or vegetables (which contain potassium).

Diarrhea Medicines

In some cases, medicines that stop diarrhea may be helpful. Diarrhea medicines that are available without a doctor's prescription include Imodium (loperamide), Pepto-Bismol, and Kaopectate. Stop taking these medicines if symptoms get worse or if your diarrhea lasts more than two days.

Doctors do not recommend using these medicines when the diarrhea is bloody or you have a fever or abdominal pain.. Stopping the diarrhea in such cases traps the organism in the intestines, prolonging the problem. Instead, doctors usually prescribe antibiotics for diarrhea treatment in these cases:

- **Bacterial infection.** Salmonella, campylobacter, E. coli and Shigella are the most common types of bacterial infection causing diarrhea in developing countries and are found in the United States as well. E. coli diarrhea is commonly called traveler's diarrhea and the most effective treatment is the use of azithromycin (z-pack) or ciprofloxacin (Cipro). These are prescription medicines.
- **Giardiasis.** Giardia usually infects people who drink water that contains the parasite. Giardiasis can last months or longer without treatment and spreads rapidly. The treatment is medication called tinidazole or metronidazole, which is a prescription medicine. Azithromycin is sometimes used in Asian missions.

PREVENTION

You usually catch infectious types of diarrhea by actually eating microscopic viruses, bacteria, or parasites. These microbes then flourish in your intestines, causing diarrhea. But how do the little creatures end up in our mouths in the first place? The answer is simple, but disgusting: the offending microbes usually are passed from the diarrhea of others. For example, it comes from drinking water that has not been treated after animals have used it for their bathroom. It also comes from those who don't wash their hands after having bowel movements. These people pass infections by preparing food, shaking hands, or touching other objects with contaminated hands.

Prevention is a matter of good hygiene.

- Always wash your hands before preparing food for yourself or for others.
- If you are in a location where you have to place used toilet paper in a container, cover the container so that flies don't land on it and spread bacteria that cause diarrhea.
- Keep your hands away from your mouth in general.
- Wash your hands after shaking hands with a number of people.
- Of course, always wash your hands after using the bathroom, and be wary of those who don't.
- Carry hand sanitizer for occasions when it is not possible for you to wash your hands. When possible, avoid potentially contaminated foods such as unwashed produce or produce that may have been washed in contaminated water.
- Drink safe water.

EAR PAIN

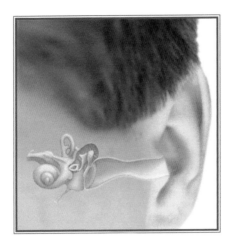

The causes of ear pain are almost too many to list, but there are some common causes that missionaries should know about. Ear pain is often caused by a buildup of fluid and pressure behind the eardrum, in the area called the middle ear. The middle ear is connected to the nasal passages by a short narrow tube, the Eustachian tube. A cold or allergy can block the Eustachian tube due to inflammation and the buildup of secretions. Then fluid will build up in the middle ear and cause pain. Trying to open the Eustachian tube will help relieve pain. Flying to your mission or to a new area might cause ear pain as well. However, ear pain may actually be coming from another location, such as your jaw joint, your teeth or your throat. Here is a short list:

- Joint pain in the jaw
- Middle ear infection - acute
- Outer ear canal infection
- From pressure changes in an airplane
- Ruptured or perforated eardrum
- Sinus infection
- Sore throat
- Tooth infection

The following steps may help an earache:

- Applying a cold pack or cold wet wash-cloth to the outer ear.
- Chewing gum to relieve the pain and pressure
- Resting in an upright position can help reduce pressure in the middle ear.
- Using over-the-counter ear drops as long as the eardrum has not ruptured.
- Taking acetaminophen/ paracemetol or ibuprofen.
- Using a decongestant and/or nasal spray to help open the Eustachian tube.

Other steps you can try:

- Tap on each tooth and see if it is a toothache causing your ear pain. If it is, you will need to work with a dentist (refer to the chapter on toothache and dental problems)
- Place your finger at the back of the jaw joint right in front of your ear and see if it hurts when you open and close your mouth. This might indicate that it is jaw pain that is really causing ear pain.
- Do you have a cold or a sinus infection? This might be causing the ear pain (refer to the chapter on colds).

When to Contact a Medical Professional

- You have a fever or severe pain
- New symptoms appear, especially:
  - Dizziness
  - Severe headache
  - Swelling around the ear
  - Weakness of the face muscles
- Symptoms get worse or do not improve within 24 - 48 hours
- A discharge from the ear is seen
- Blood from the ear is seen

EYE PROBLEMS

CONJUNCTIVITIS (PINKEYE)

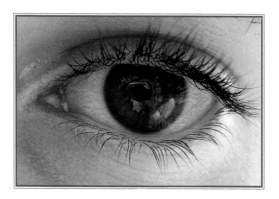

Conjunctivitis is inflammation of the membrane that covers the white of the eye. When this layer of the eye becomes inflamed the eyes will appear bloodshot, produce tears, and sometimes even swell. They often itch and are irritated. The infected and irritated membrane can produce pus, causing the eyelids to stick together after they have been closed. If this is the case, carefully splash them with some lukewarm water to loosen any "gunk" so you can open them.

Conjunctivitis is most often caused by viruses, bacteria, allergies, or chemical irritants (makeup, contact lens solutions, and dust). Conjunctivitis is most frequently caused by viruses. Viral conjunctivitis is VERY contagious. It may start in one eye and then spread to the other. Be careful after washing and drying your face – don't let anyone else use that towel, as it is contagious. It often spreads from one missionary to another. Make sure you wash your hands after touching or rubbing your eyes. Viral conjunctivitis will typically resolve in 7 to 14 days.

Although much less frequent, bacterial conjunctivitis can lead to a sight-threatening injury. Often it progresses more rapidly, produces more pus and affects vision by causing clouding of the cornea (the clear center portion of the eye). Wearing your contact lenses for too long or overnight may increase your risk for bacterial conjunctivitis.

Conjunctivitis that is associated with allergies almost always affects both eyes and is often associated with an "itchy" sensation. You may notice that your eyes are more affected at different times of the year. It may be treated with prescription eye drops. Allergic conjunctivitis is not contagious and is often worse in the morning. It may be treated with prescription eye drops.

Treatment

If you wear contact lenses, stop wearing them and use your prescription glasses. There are over-the-counter and prescription eye drops that may reduce your symptoms. If you think you have viral or bacterial conjunctivitis, call the mission office or doctor who can prescribe eye drops to make you more comfortable.

SCRATCHED EYE

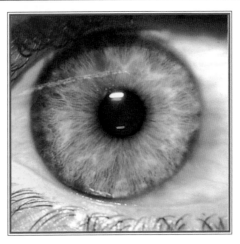

If the front of the eye is damaged, the eye becomes inflamed and there can be significant pain and tearing. A scratch on the eye can be caused by walking through tall bushes or trees. Sometimes dirt or sand can get into your eye, causing small scratches on the surface of the eye.

Treatment

Rinse your eye out with clean water. Be sure to gently rinse under your eyelids to make sure that there is no remaining foreign material trapped beneath. Even after cleaning the eye, you may feel like there is still "sand" there – this often happens when the surface of the eye has been scratched. Call the mission doctor right away if you do get a scratch like this on the surface of the eyeball. An infection can occur from the scratch. You will be given prescription eye drops and sometimes oral medication to prevent infection. The eye can heal very quickly, but you must seek attention quickly with this kind of injury.

EYESTRAIN

Eyestrain causes a dull, aching sensation around and behind the eyes that can progress into a generalized headache. It may feel painful or fatiguing to focus the eyes. Eyestrain is commonly a result of overuse of the eyes for activities requiring close and precise focus, such as reading and using the computer. This has become a common problem for missionaries who study a lot.

Treatment

Lie down, close your eyes, and place a cold compress or ice pack on your eyes. Relax your eyes for at least ten minutes. Try to avoid eyestrain by taking periodic "focus breaks." About every twenty minutes, try to look away from your work and focus on something in the distance for a minute or two. Getting enough sleep can also help.

DRY EYES

It is common for people who spend a lot of time reading or looking at computer screens to get dry eyes. Remember to blink and take occasional breaks.

Treatment

An over-the-counter eye drop can help relieve such symptoms.

STY

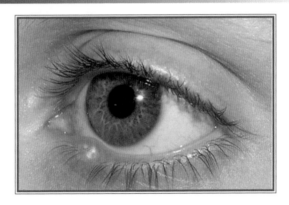

A sty is a bacterial infection within a gland on the edge of the eyelid. The sty takes on the appearance of a small pimple and can become inflamed and tender. The sty will gradually come to a head, open, and drain.

Treatment

Apply a warm compress or a warm, damp cloth and gently massage the area for about ten minutes. This will help relieve discomfort and bring the sty to a head so that it can drain and healing can begin. In stubborn cases, you may need to be treated with antibiotics. Call the mission doctor for further instructions or to see if he or she wants to prescribe an antibiotic for you.

SERIOUS EYE PROBLEMS

There are a handful of emergencies associated with the eye. If you have any of the following symptoms, you should seek medical attention as soon as possible:

- Sudden loss of vision in all or part of your field of vision
- Sudden appearance of flashes of light or floaters in your field of vision

FATIGUE AND SLEEPINESS

A common complaint among missionaries is feeling tired. Some missionaries may fall asleep while studying or teaching. When missionaries say they are sleepy, they usually mean that they are fatigued. Fatigue is different from sleepiness. Sleepiness is simply feeling the need to fall asleep. Fatigue, on the other hand, is a general lack of energy and motivation.

There are many possible physical and psychological causes of fatigue. Fatigue can be a response to physical exertion or to stress, or it can be caused by a lack of sleep. In addition in some countries, some viruses such as the Epstein-Barr or CMV may cause fatigue. These can be detected by a physician. Some other common causes include:

- Allergies
- Medicines (such as antihistamines)
- Depression or stress
- Persistent pain
- Lack of sleep
- Dehydration
- Poor diets that are high in sugar and low in nutrients
- Hot and humid weather

Some tips for reducing fatigue are:

- Try to get adequate amounts of sleep each night.
- Eat a healthy, well-balanced diet and drink plenty of water throughout the day.

- Add more fruits and vegetables to your diet.
- If you can't get enough nutritious food during the week, take a multivitamin.
- Exercise the required 30 minutes each day.

Fatigue can be caused by more serious conditions such as thyroid problems or anemia. If the above suggestions don't help your fatigue, make sure you talk with the mission doctor.

FLEAS/BEDBUGS

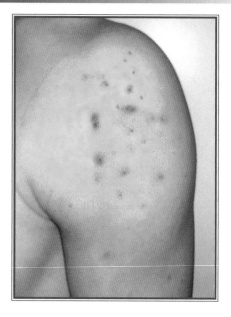

Missionaries can encounter fleas and bedbugs in all missions, but fleas are particularly prevalent in developing countries. Also both are becoming more common in the United States. Most flea bites occur around the ankles and legs but can occur anywhere on the body. Fleas and bedbugs live in mattresses and bite the missionary at night. Depending upon a person's sensitivity, the irritation from the bites may last from a few minutes to a few hours or even days. The typical flea bite may appear as a small, hard, red, itchy area. There is a single puncture point in the center of the red spot. Symptoms often begin suddenly within hours.

HOW IT IS SPREAD

Fleas lay eggs on humans, dogs, cats, and other animals. Flea larvae emerge from the eggs to feed on dead skin, feces, and vegetable matter. The adult flea can stay dormant for weeks until a host is near and then the flea jumps or crawls onto the new host, where it can lay new eggs and continue its life cycle.

TREATMENT

Do not scratch the affected area! This can prolong the healing time. Wash the bites with antiseptic lotion or soap. Use cold water – warm or hot water may worsen the itch. The itching associated with flea bites can be treated with anti-itch creams (usually antihistamines or hydrocortisone). Calamine lotion has been shown to be ineffective for itching caused by bedbugs and fleas.

Oral doses of antihistamines such as Dimetapp, Chlor-Trimeton, and Benadryl may also relieve itching and swelling.

PREVENTION

Cleanliness is key to fighting fleas. Also, you can try to lower the humidity and temperature in your apartment. Vacuuming can eliminate fleas from an apartment. Altering even one of these environmental factors may be enough to drastically lower and eliminate an infestation. Look for little spots of blood on your sheets when you get up in the morning. This is likely from a flea bite. Washing sheets and getting a new mattress, if possible, well help as well.

The best preventative measure is to avoid animals or bedding that are known to have fleas. If this is not possible, you can soak bedding or clothes in a synthetic chemical called permethrin. It is harmless to humans but usually kills fleas (and other insects) instantly on contact. See the appendix on permethrin for more information. Putting flea collars around the bed posts may also help.

FROSTBITE
AND FROSTNIP

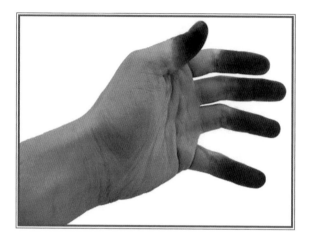

Many missionaries serve in areas of the world where temperatures may drop well below freezing, making them susceptible to cold injuries. The common pain that most people
experience in their fingers, toes, or face during and after cold
exposure is called frostnip, which consists of near-freezing
of tissues. Frostbite is more severe and involves formation of
ice in body tissues. Missionaries working in cold temperatures should be familiar with frostbite and frostnip to avoid
not only pain and discomfort, but also more serious tissue
damage.

FROSTNIP

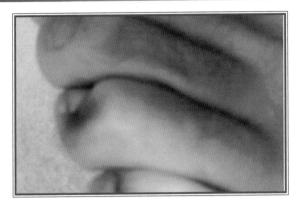

Most people experience some degree of frostnip when exposed to the cold. The extremities, such as the fingers, toes, earlobes, and tip of the nose are most likely to be affected by frostnip because the body decreases circulation to these areas in low temperatures. It is important to realize that factors such as wind and moisture can induce frostnip even when temperatures are well above freezing.

Diagnosis

Depending on the severity, your skin may appear red due to the initial inflammation or pale due to decreasing circulation. Frostnip victims will experience pain and/or numbness in the affected area. Upon re-warming, sensation returns with pain that will initially intensify before it subsides.

Treatment

The most effective treatment is rapid rewarming to avoid development of frostbite. If warm water is available, rewarm 15-30 minutes at a temperature of 104-108°F (40-42.2°C), approximately spa temperature. This is usually painful. If warm water is not readily available, other methods are: covering your nose or ears with warm hands, blowing warm air over your hands, and placing your hands in your armpits or near some other heat source. Because wind and water can aggravate the cold, remove wet clothing and cover yourself with warm, dry clothing or blankets. Do not rub area or gradually rewarm with cold, then hotter water. Both of these methods increase the danger of tissue damage.

FROSTBITE

Frostbite is localized tissue freezing that occurs because of exposure to freezing or near-freezing temperatures. In extreme circumstances, skin can freeze in a matter of minutes or even seconds. Wind and water contribute significantly to cooling, and frostbite can occur above freezing temperatures if a person is wearing wet clothing on a windy day. Repeated frostbiting of an area can severely damage tissues. For this reason, only rewarm an area when there is no longer a risk of refreezing.

Diagnosis

Frostbite presents itself with pain or numbness and discoloration. Based on the severity, the tissues may range from blotchy yellow-white to pale white with a solid "chunk of wood" texture. Upon re-warming, severely frostbitten tissues will develop blisters that may be filled with clear fluid or blood.

Treatment

Rapidly rewarm the affected part for 15-30 minutes in water at a temperature of 104-108°F (40-42.2°C) as is the case with frostnip. Again, this is a painful process. If there is any risk of refreezing the area, wait to rewarm. Do not rewarm using dry heat such as fire to avoid burning the frostbitten skin. Take anti-inflammatory medication (like ibuprofen) to alleviate the pain and inflammation associated with re-warming. Consult your mission doctor in any case of frostbite.

PREVENTION OF FROSTNIP AND FROSTBITE

- Do not go outside in very cold weather after a recent bath or shower.
- Wear warm, dry clothing and dress in loose layers.
- Wear hats, scarves, gloves, mittens, and well-fitted, waterproof boots.
- Keep dry. Change quickly out of wet clothing.

FUNGAL INFECTIONS

Fungal infections of the skin are very common among missionaries. Fungal infections are contagious. Sometimes people get a fungal infection from direct contact with an infected person. A fungal infection also can be picked up by touching an infected pet or item contaminated with the fungus. Fungi thrive in warm, moist areas. A comb, clothing, or shower surface can all harbor fungi.

Athlete's Foot

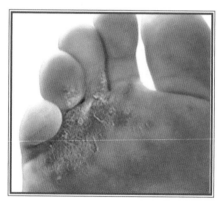

Athlete's foot is a very common fungal infection. It is spread by touching your foot to an area where the fungus is found, such as on a bathroom floor or bathtub. Athlete's foot begins between the toes. It is here that the skin peels, cracks, and scales. Itching is common. Redness, scaling, and dryness can develop on the soles and along the sides of the feet. For mild cases of athlete's foot, antifungal creams are effective and can relieve symptoms such as burning and itching.

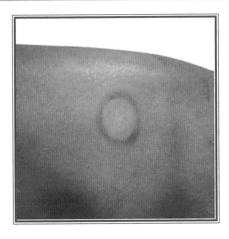

Ringworm

Ringworm is a contagious fungal infection that is usually spread from person to person. Ringworm appears on the skin as an itchy, red, scaly patch that is ring-shaped.

Jock Itch

Jock itch is a rash that develops in the groin and buttocks area and affects both men and women. Individuals who tend to sweat a lot may be more susceptible to jock itch. The rash is itchy, has a red border, and can spread.

PREVENTION AND TREATMENT

Poor hygiene and prolonged wet skin increase the risk of developing a fungal infection. Most fungal infections will get better with simple hygiene principles.

- Wash the affected area daily. Dry the skin carefully after bathing.
- Wash towels often.

- Apply antifungal cream or powder three times daily.
- Do not urinate on the fungal infection while taking a shower. That does not work and might make it worse.

Athlete's foot (foot infection)

- Wear flip-flops in changing areas.
- Use antifungal sprays or powders in shoes.
- After a shower, dry your feet and between your toes last to prevent spread to other parts of the skin.
- Avoid tight or closed footwear, especially in warm climates.
- Change socks daily.
- Do not wear your companion's or anyone else's shoes.
- Wear cotton or synthetic sweat socks to absorb perspiration.

Jock itch (groin infection)

- After a shower, dry your groin before drying your feet to reduce the risk of spreading fungus from your feet.
- Change underwear daily.

Ringworm (skin infection)

- Ringworm on the body can either spread from fungus elsewhere on the skin or from contact with others.

Antifungal medicines are best applied two to three times daily. If one does not work, try another brand as it might be more effective. You can get over-the-counter antifungal products in a variety of forms, such as cream, lotion, powder, and spray. Cream and lotion antifungal products are preferred for ringworm infections on the body. Common over-the-counter antifungals are tolnaftate (Tinactin), clotrimazole (Lotrimin), and miconazole (Micatin). Powder and spray products are more suitable for athlete's foot. Apply these products to the affected area twice daily for at least four weeks.

HEADACHES

Headache is a term used to describe aching or pain that occurs in one or more areas of the head, face, mouth, or neck. Headaches are common among missionaries. Headaches can be chronic, recurrent, or occasional. The pain can be mild or severe enough to disrupt daily activities.

Tension Headache

About 90% of headaches among missionaries are tension headaches. Tension headaches are usually caused by the layer of muscle around the skull contracting, which in turn can decrease blood flow to your head. This causes a band of pressure/pain around your head. Sometimes it's a constant pain, and other times it's more of a throbbing pain. In any case, this type of headache is not serious or dangerous, but it is very uncomfortable.

Sinus Headache

A sinus headache is caused by an infection or inflammation in your sinuses. This causes a buildup of pressure, which results in a dull, aching pain usually experienced at the upper part of the nose and under the eyes. It may start on one side, but may spread to both sides as the infection and inflammation get worse. Lying down often makes the pain worse. You may also have other symptoms such as congestion, fever, and fatigue. People with a deviated septum (the tissue in between nostrils is sometimes bent) may get this type of headache more often.

Cluster Headache

Cluster headaches are another type of headache that is typically very painful. They are usually only on one side and are described as sharp or boring pain behind the eye or in the temple, sometimes radiating to the neck. They can last for minutes to hours and usually come in clusters, hence the name. For example, someone may go for months without any headache, and then have several over a few days. Overall, they are very rare. The cause of cluster headaches is somewhat of a mystery.

Migraine

This type of headache can be very severe and often has several parts to it. People who experience migraines often experience symptoms before the actual headache arrives, such as a change in mood, cravings for certain foods, tense muscles, increased urge to urinate, or other things. There can also be something called an aura phase. This usually occurs minutes to hours before the onset of a headache and most often includes visual changes such as blurriness, flashing lights, or even temporary loss of vision in one eye. Some people also experience numbness and tingling in their hands, arms, mouth, and even tongue. The headache is usually on one side, and the pain is usually described as moderate to severe and sometimes throbbing pain. People may also be nauseated, and can be extremely sensitive to light and sound. Migraine headaches usually last from several hours up to a few days. There can be a phase after the headache where you experience fatigue, weakness, diarrhea or constipation, or other symptoms. The cause of migraine headaches is still a mystery.

TREATMENT

Treatment depends on the type, the severity, and the frequency of occurrence of your headache.

Tension headaches usually can be treated successfully with lifestyle adjustments and over-the-counter pain medicines such as aspirin, ibuprofen, and acetaminophen / paracetamol. Symptoms from sinus headaches can also sometimes be treated with these types of over-the-counter medicines. But, if there is a significant sinus infection, antibiotics may be required.

Cluster and migraine type headaches tend to be much more severe and may require prescription medications and preventative treatment. Most missionaries who have cluster or migraine headaches are aware of this before coming into the mission field. If your headaches are not better with treatment, or if they worsen, be sure to see the mission doctor.

Note: If you have headaches that are associated with a stiff neck or if light makes your eyes hurt you should contact the mission president or mission doctor.

HEMORRHOIDS
(Sores in the Rectum)

DESCRIPTION

If you noticed blood on the toilet paper, you likely have what is called a hemorrhoid. A burning feeling when you go to the bathroom is also suggestive of a hemorrhoid. Hemorrhoids are abnormally swollen veins in the area where you go to the bathroom. Some are high up (internal hemorrhoids) and some are down low (external hemorrhoids). These areas are called the rectum and anus. Hemorrhoids are caused by too much pressure in the rectum often from hard stools and constipation. They can also be caused by excessive straining during bowel movements, heavy coughing, or heavy lifting.

TREATMENT AND PREVENTION

It is important to identify the cause of your hemorrhoids. Once you have eliminated factors causing your hemorrhoids, you can begin treating them. There are two goals of treatment. The first is to treat the symptoms, including the burning, the pain, and the itching. The second is to shrink the hemorrhoids.

- Over-the-counter pain medicine such as acetaminophen / paracetamol, ibuprofen, or Aleve (naproxen) can be used for the aching pain.
- The burning and itching responds best to steroid creams and suppositories. These medicines are also very helpful in shrinking the hemorrhoids.
- It is also important to cleanse the entire rectal area with warm water after each bowel movement.

- Using a bulk fiber laxative such as methyl cellulose (Citrucel) or psyllium fiber (Metamucil) will help soften stools. This can help eliminate straining with bowel movements. Remember, bulk fiber may take several days to work, but, when used on a regular basis, can be very effective at preventing recurrence.
- Rarely, surgery is required to remove the hemorrhoids.

RECOMMENDED PRODUCTS

- Aleve (naproxen), ibuprofen, or Tylenol (acetaminophen / paracetamol). Use these quick-acting anti-inflammatory medications for the aching discomfort of severe hemorrhoidal flare ups.
- Anusol HC cream (hydrocortisone 1%). For swollen external hemorrhoids, brands containing hydrocortisone such as this one are effective at reducing the swelling, burning, and itching sensations.
- Anusol HC suppositories (hydrocortisone 1% suppositories). These hydrocortisone suppositories should be used for internal swelling and discomfort.
- Citrucel (methylcellulose, 2 grams/Tbs). Softening stools and treating constipation are crucial aspects of treating your hemorrhoids. Many find this brand of bulk fiber laxative to be less gritty than others, and it comes in both sugared and sugar-free versions. Any bulk fiber will work.

HIGH ALTITUDE SICKNESS

Many missionaries who travel to high altitudes are unaware that elevation change can cause illnesses. High altitude sickness tends to occur in people above 8,000 feet (2,500 meters) in elevation. The higher in altitude, the more likely people will become ill. Is your mission high in altitude? If so then you may be at risk for altitude illness. As we go up in altitude there is less atmospheric pressure as well as less breathable oxygen. This leads to shortness of breath even when doing normal tasks (i.e. walking up stairs, exercising), headache, dizziness, and fatigue. Something that is important to note with high altitude sickness is the fact that it is unpredictable. Even very healthy and fit people can suffer from high altitude sickness. There are three different diseases that can occur at altitude. These are acute mountain illness (AMS), high altitude cerebral edema (HACE), and high altitude pulmonary edema (HAPE).

AMS: Acute Mountain Illness is the most common of the three. It is caused by mild brain swelling. Symptoms can be subtle or severe. Usually people will have a headache but often will have one or more of the following as well:

- Nausea or vomiting
- Loss of appetite
- General weakness
- Dizziness
- Trouble sleeping (Insomnia)
- Malaise
- Diarrhea (sometimes constipation)
- Light headedness

HACE: AMS can progress to High Altitude Cerebral Edema (HACE) which is much more serious and even potentially fatal. HACE is when the brain continues to swell within the skull due to low oxygen pressure. Symptoms of High Altitude Cerebral Edema are:

- Headache that does not respond to painkillers
- Unsteady gait and poor coordination
- Confusion or gradual loss of consciousness
- Increased nausea
- Difficulty seeing things

HAPE: Another major illness that can happen at the same time, and not directly related to AMS or HACE, is called High Altitude Pulmonary Edema (HAPE). This is when fluid gathers in the lungs due to pressure changes. This is a dangerous and possibly fatal disease. Symptoms of HAPE are:

- Symptoms similar to bronchitis
- Persistent cough often with wet sputum
- Fever
- Shortness of breath even when resting

TREATMENT

If you are in a mission and you were transferred to an area that is high in altitude and have any of these symptoms (particularly a headache or shortness of breath) you may well have altitude illness. The best treatment for any high altitude sickness is quick descent to a lower altitude. You need to talk to the mission president or the mission doctor, and ask to be moved to a lower elevation quickly. For HAPE and HACE and for more severe forms of AMS, rapid decent is important. Dropping in elevation has instant positive effects and usually leads to instant recovery. If you feel sick and can't get down, hospitals often have supplemental oxygen. This can also provide great relief. In some areas where high altitude sickness is known to be a common problem, hospitals may also be equipped with a hyperbaric chamber. A hyperbaric chamber's main function is to simulate a drop in elevation by increasing the pressure to that of about sea level. This increase in pressure along with an increase in oxygen levels within the chamber help to relieve and even cure high altitude sickness. Even though there are treatments that will help to decrease the symptoms of high altitude sickness no treatment can rival the effectiveness of descent. It is highly recommended that rapid descent be performed before all other treatments, especially if diagnosed with HAPE or HACE.

PREVENTION

The best way to avoid getting high altitude sickness is to travel slowly to an area that is very high. This might be hard to do on a transfer. In that case, take it easy when you get to altitude. Rest and relax to allow your body to become accustomed to the effects of altitude. Avoid exercise and walk slowly up stairs and ramps for the first few days. Learn to sit down if you become short of breath. In time, usually over several days, your body will change to handle the effects of altitude better. Remember to stay very hydrated. Fluid is essential in preventing high altitude illness. Some places will have you drink various drinks such as coca tea or gingko biloba. These may be useful but it is more important that you stay well hydrated.

INFLUENZA

Influenza (the flu) is a contagious respiratory illness caused by the influenza viruses. These viruses most often circulate in the winter in temperate climates but can also occur in tropical climates. Influenza can cause mild to severe illness.

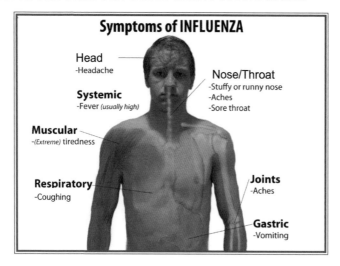

Symptoms of influenza usually start quite suddenly, one to two days after exposure. Usually the first symptoms are fever, which can make you feel either hot or cold (chills) with body temperatures ranging from 38-39°C (approximately 100-103°F). Many people are so ill that they are confined to bed for several days with aches and pains throughout their bodies, which are worse in their back and legs. Other symptoms of influenza may include:

- Fatigue and body aches, especially joints
- Sore throat

- Cough and congestion
- Headache
- Irritated watering eyes

It can be difficult to distinguish between the common cold and influenza in the early stages of these infections, but flu can be identified by *a high fever with a sudden onset and extreme fatigue*. Influenza's effects are much more severe and last longer than those of the common cold. Most people will recover completely in about one to two weeks. Diarrhea is not normally a symptom of influenza in adults, but it can be on occasion.

CAUSES

People who contract influenza are most likely to pass it to others during the time period between when symptoms begin and around ten days after that. Influenza can be spread in three main ways: 1) when an infected person sneezes mucus into the eyes, nose or mouth of another person; 2) when people inhale the aerosols produced by infected people coughing or sneezing; and 3) through hand-to-mouth transmission such as a handshake. Missionaries shake a lot of hands. This is one more reason to wash your hands frequently.

TREATMENT

Missionaries with the flu are advised to get plenty of rest and drink plenty of liquids. Some medicines that might help to relieve the fever and muscle aches associated with the flu are:

- Paracetamol / acetaminophen (Tylenol)
- Ibuprofen (Advil)

Note: You should *not* take aspirin to treat the flu.

Since influenza is caused by a virus, antibiotics have no effect on the infection; unless they are prescribed for secondary infections such as bacterial pneumonia.

The antiviral drugs oseltamivir (Tamiflu) and zanamivir (Relenza) can be effective but should only be used if recommended by a physician. Other antiviral drugs such as amantadine and rimantadine are also sometimes used. A prescription will be needed for these.

PREVENTION

Good personal health and hygiene habits, like hand washing, avoiding spitting, and covering the nose and mouth (with your upper sleeve, not your hand) when sneezing or coughing, are reasonably effective in reducing influenza transmission. In particular, frequent hand washing with soap and water, or with alcohol-based hand rubs, is very effective at inactivating influenza viruses.

INGROWN TOENAIL

DESCRIPTION

Since missionaries spend a lot of time on their feet, they are prone to develop ingrown toenails. An ingrown toenail curves downward and grows into the skin, usually at the sides of the nail. As it digs in, the nail irritates the skin causing pain, redness, swelling, and a hot sensation in the toe. The warm, moist skin inside your shoe is a perfect environment for bacteria to grow. If an ingrown nail breaks the skin, bacteria can enter and cause an infection, which may result in pus and a foul odor.

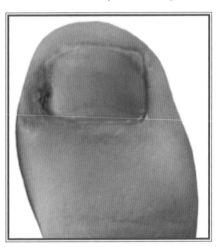

CAUSES

Ingrown toenails can develop for various reasons. Some missionaries may develop an ingrown toenail much more easily due to their inherited foot shape. But they are usually caused by excessive pressure on the toe from long hours on the feet walking, from running, or from trauma such as a stubbed toe.

When missionaries neglect proper foot care, the risk of ingrown toenails is greatly increased. Trimming nails too short or too curved on the outer edges encourages the nail to dig into skin. Shoes that do not fit properly press the toenail into the skin as well.

TREATMENT

Sometimes initial treatment for ingrown toenails can be safely performed at home. However, home treatment is strongly discouraged if you suspect you have an infection, or if you have a medical condition that puts your feet at high risk such as diabetes or poor blood circulation in the foot.

- **Home care.** If you don't have an infection or any of the above conditions, you can soak your foot in warm water (add Epsom salt if you wish), and gently massage the side of the nail fold while lightly elevating the corners of the nail. Do this twice daily to relieve skin irritation and inflammation.

Avoid attempting "bathroom surgery." Repeated cutting of the nail or attempts to elevate the corners of the nail after they have broken the skin can cause the condition to worsen over time. If you develop an infection or your symptoms fail to improve, it's time to see a foot doctor, who will probably recommend the following treatments:

- **Oral antibiotics.** If an infection is present, an oral antibiotic may be prescribed.
- **Surgery.** A simple procedure, often performed in the office, is commonly needed to ease the pain and remove the offending nail. Surgery may involve numbing the toe and removing a corner of the nail, a larger portion of the nail, or the entire nail.

PREVENTION

Many cases of ingrown toenails may be prevented by following these two important tips:

- **Trim your nails properly.** Don't cut them too short – making sure you can slip the end of your fingernail under the corner of the toenail. Cut toenails in a straight line so that the curved edges don't dig in. If your toenails curve steeply at the corners, do not dig away at folds – seek professional help.
- **Avoid poorly fitting shoes.** Wear a shoe that holds your foot snugly without sliding around but also allows enough room in the toe box for you to wiggle your toes. Wear sandals or loose slippers while you are at home as often as needed.

INSOMNIA

It is very important to sleep at night. If a missionary does not sleep well, it will show in poor mental functioning the next day. Insomnia is difficulty falling asleep or staying asleep. It is often a symptom of stress, depression or anxiety.

Sometimes insomnia will be for just a few nights such as when you move to a new country, move to a new time zone or move to a new area with a different bed and new sleeping conditions. In these cases the insomnia should only last for a few days or for a few weeks.

However, if the insomnia persists, then it can be caused by a psychological problem such as stress, anxiety, or depession. All of these are common among missionaries. (Refer to the chapters on depression and anxiety.)

TREATMENT

It is important to get help for insomnia if it does not get better on its own. Speak to the mission president or the mission doctor in this case. If stress, anxiety, or depression is the problem, then talking with someone may help.

Sometimes medicines will be helpful. The most effective medical treatments for insomnia are prescription drugs. However, there are a number of over-the-counter medications that will help as well. These are antihistamines. Any antihistamine will work but the most common ones are Benadryl, Dimetapp, Chlor-Trimeton, and Tylenol PM.

MALARIA

Missionaries in many parts of the world are at risk for contracting malaria. It is one of the most pervasive diseases in the world. Symptoms of malaria include fever, shivering, joint pain, vomiting, anemia, reddish urine, retinal damage, and convulsions. The classic symptom of malaria is cyclical occurrence of sudden coldness followed by shaking and then fever and sweating lasting four to six hours, occurring every two days.

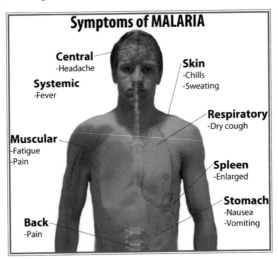

Symptoms of MALARIA

Central
-Headache

Systemic
-Fever

Skin
-Chills
-Sweating

Respiratory
-Dry cough

Muscular
-Fatigue
-Pain

Spleen
-Enlarged

Stomach
-Nausea
-Vomiting

Back
-Pain

HOW IT IS SPREAD

- Malaria is spread by mosquitos.
- The disease is acquired when a mosquito bites an infected carrier then passes it on to a new host.

- Symptoms can appear from several weeks to several months after the malaria parasite is passed on by a mosquito bite.

TREATMENT

- If you suspect you have contracted malaria, contact your mission doctor.
- Treatment of malaria involves supportive measures as well as specific anti-malarial drugs.
- When properly treated, someone with malaria can expect a complete recovery.

PREVENTION

- In missions where malaria is a problem, the Church will provide the outline for pills to take to help prevent this disease. Make sure you take these pills – they work to give partial immunity to someone infected with this disease. Some missionaries don't like to take them for various reasons. But it is important that you do.
- Don't rely on medicines to prevent this disease. You must take steps to prevent mosquito bites in the first place.
  - You should use DEET on your skin, sleep under nets at nights, and apply permethrin to your clothes, bedding material and nets.
  - You can also hang mosquito netting over the windows or you can just hang the net in your room to help keep mosquitos away.

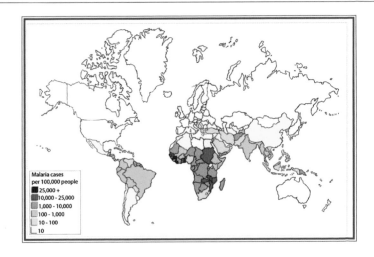

POISON IVY

Poison Ivy: demonstrating the classical "leaves of three" appearance

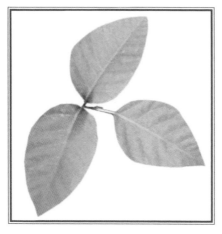

Poison Oak: with serrated edges easily confused with typical oak

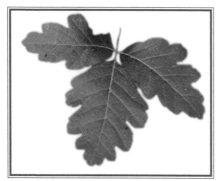

Poison Sumac: this deceptively attractive shrub is most commonly found in swampy regions

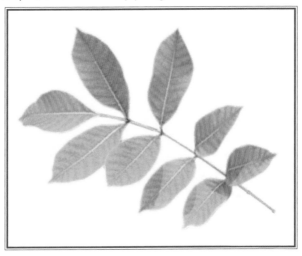

POISON IVY RASH

Missionaries might encounter plants that cause a rash. The pictures above show the three most common plants in North America that contain the toxin urishiol. Urishiol is contained in the leaves, fruit, root, and stem of these plants and can cause an itchy rash when it comes in contact with human skin. Urishiol is also very resilient and can stick to a pet, tool, or clothing and cause irritation even years after the plant was touched. As a missionary, you should be aware of these plants because of the amount of time you spend walking on roads and pathways.

- Poison ivy is a vine that can lay low on the forest floor or climb up walls and trees and is recognizable by its characteristic three leaves.
- Poison oak has a three-leaf appearance similar to poison ivy. However, its leaves are not smooth but rather serrated like typical oak leaves.
- Poison sumac has many leaves and is most common in swampy regions.

PREVENTION

Rashes are most common when urishiol is rubbed directly on the skin. Long clothing helps to protect against exposure, but urishiol can still soak through clothing and cause irritation. The surest way to avoid urishiol exposure is to recognize these toxic plants and avoid them.

TREATMENT

Early Treatment

Though a rash usually develops in 24 to 48 hours, most irritations from urishiol exposure will resolve in one to three weeks without treatment, but they can be painful and uncomfortable. The following will help in alleviating pain and minimizing irritation:

- Washing the area gently with large amounts of cold water and mild hand soap within 1-4 hours can prevent a reaction.
- Rubbing alcohol is also very effective at removing resin from skin or clothing. To avoid spreading urishiol, do not reuse cotton swabs or paper towels.
- Take care to remove resin from fingernails.

Mild Rash

Mild exposure to urishiol will result in small eruptions of rash or irritated skin and fluid-filled vesicles. The most notable symptom will be itching in the affected area. If available, high strength topical steroid creams like Zanfel or an equivalent can help relieve and blunt the allergic reaction to urishiol. These medicines will remove the toxin on the skin and relieve itching quickly.

Once blisters form, few treatments are effective to lessen the rash, but the following treatments aid in itch relief:

- Oral antihistamines or Benadryl
- Topical steroid cream (Zanfel)
- Calamine lotion
- Aveeno oatmeal baths
- Burrow's solution or Domeboro astringent solution for dried vesicles

Moderate Rash

Moderate rashes result from larger exposure, cover a larger body surface area and cause significant distress. As in mild exposure, Zanfel or other topical steroid creams can help reduce the rash before vesicle formation. After blisters form, your mission doctor can give prednisone for greater relief.

Severe Rash

Any reaction that results in swelling of the airway or genitals, or that covers a larger body surface area should be considered severe. In this case, talk to the mission doctor. You will need to take oral steroids for this. Often they will give you prednisone, which is an effective method for getting rid of the rash and the itch.

RASH

Many missionaries will develop a rash sometime while on their mission. Although rashes are seldom dangerous, as a general rule, self-diagnosis is not usually a good idea. Proper evaluation of a skin rash requires a visit to a doctor or other healthcare professional. However, missionaries may find themselves in a situation where medical care is not available. There might be some things you can do if you are not near someone with medical experience. This chapter will get you started. The term 'rash' can refer to many different skin conditions. Common categories of rashes and how to treat them are listed below.

SCALY PATCHES OF SKIN CAUSED BY A FUNGUS OR A BACTERIAL INFECTION

Fungus is a common cause of a red, scaly skin rash. These include ringworm, athlete's foot and jock itch. If you suspect a fungal infection, use the procedures outlined in the fungal infections chapter.

Many bacterial skin infections need to be treated with antibiotics. Bacterial skin infections are often associated with a cut or a puncture in the skin, but sometimes these are hard to see. They tend to spread rapidly. They can be wet and weeping and can burn, itch, or be painful. Minor bacterial skin infections may be treated simply by using topical antibiotic ointment like Neosporin. However, some more serious infections can progress and make you feel generally sick. In this case you should see a doctor and/or call the mission doctor as you might need oral antibiotics in addition to topical antibiotics.

SCALY PATCHES OF SKIN NOT CAUSED BY INFECTIONS CALLED ECZEMA

Scaly, itchy skin patches often represent one of the conditions referred to as eczema. This is often a hereditary skin problem that missionaries will already know about. Eczema comes and goes on its own schedule, unlike allergy-related rashes that are associated with foods, soaps, or detergents. In most cases of eczema, changing your diet or detergent does not help the rash.

Eczema is often worse in the winter months when the air is cold and dry. Frequent washing may irritate the skin and aggravate the condition.

Skin affected by eczema can become extremely itchy and inflamed. It may look red, swollen, and cracked. In some cases, the skin can also weep and crust. Liquid that oozes out of such crusts is often not infected; what comes out is the body's normal tissue fluid. This rash is not contagious.

Treatment of eczema involves minimizing irritation and the use of 1% hydrocortisone cream that can be purchased over-the-counter. Rub it on three times daily. Regularly applying moisturizing lotions, especially after bathing, can also help control your eczema.

ALLERGIC SKIN REACTION

This is a rash that is brought on either by contact with a specific material that causes a skin allergy or by something that irritates the skin, like too-frequent hand washing. Some common causes of allergic rashes include poison ivy, detergents, and metals. Allergic rashes will often be located where the allergy-inducing material (or allergen) has contacted the skin.

Treatment of an allergic skin reaction involves avoiding the allergen that caused it, if there is one, or minimizing whatever exposure is irritating the skin (e.g. water on the hands, solvents while cleaning, or saliva around the mouth from lip licking).

Effective treatments include 1% hydrocortisone and many prescription-strength creams. The cream should be applied three times daily if possible. For details about treating a poison ivy rash, see the chapter on poison ivy.

GENERAL GUIDELINES

If a rash really bothers you, contact the mission doctor.

The longer you've had a rash, the more likely it is that you need to see the mission doctor.

If you've had the same rash before, it's probably the same diagnosis.

Signs that should send you to the mission doctor sooner rather than later are:

- Pain
- Rapid swelling
- Bleeding, blisters
- Rash in the mouth or eyes
- Skin that is rapidly turning dusky or black.

SORE THROAT

Missionaries frequently get sore throats. There are many different causes of sore throats. Some require antibiotics for treatment while some cannot be treated at all, and you will just have to wait for the body to heal itself. However, over-the-counter medicines such as ibuprofen can help relieve the pain of a sore throat even if there is no "treatment." Here are some general guidelines.

SORE THROAT DUE TO COUGHS, COLDS, AND RUNNY NOSES

Coughing by itself can make your throat feel sore. So can postnasal drip, which is mucus from the nose dripping down the back of the throat.

If you have a dry cough (meaning nothing comes up when you cough), cough suppressants – some of which you can buy without a prescription – can quiet the cough and cut down on throat irritation. If you are coughing because of postnasal drip, decongestants can help reduce the postnasal drip and thus reduce the cough. However, with viral colds, decongestants may not help very much. Humidity and drinking fluids will help, since they will keep the mucus from getting thick. Thick mucus is much harder to cough out than thin mucus.

SORE THROAT DUE TO VIRUSES

Viral sore throats are very common. Many missionaries get viral sore throats because of the number of people with whom they come in contact. There are many viruses that attack the mucus membranes of the throat, the tonsils, or both. These viruses will often make your throat feel sore. Some of these viruses, like the adenoviruses, will also cause pus to accumulate on the tonsils just like strep throat does, and testing needs to be done to see whether strep is the problem. Since there are no antibiotics for viruses, you need to wait until the body gets rid of the virus on its own, which usually takes 7-10 days. Humidity and fluids will soothe the throat and acetaminophen (Tylenol) / paracetamol will help with the pain.

STREP THROAT

Although there are other bacteria that can attack the throat, the most common bacterial cause is Streptococcus pyogenes, or "strep throat." The classic strep throat is very red. Often your tonsils will be swollen and will have white or grey patches on them. You may also see little dark-red, almost purple, spots on the back of the roof of the mouth. The tongue may be very red with little white spots – a condition called a "strawberry tongue."

Usually a person with strep throat will have swollen and tender lymph nodes at the front or sides of the neck, and the throat will hurt so much that even swallowing liquids is painful. Coughing and runny nose are *rare* with strep throat, and temperature may go up to 103°F/39.5°C or more.

Fortunately, strep throats are very easy to treat. Penicillin usually works just fine, but it has to be given 4 times a day on an empty stomach. Amoxicillin also works well on strep. It can be given three times a day, and it doesn't matter much if you give it on a full or an empty stomach. If you are allergic to penicillin there are other antibiotics that you can take. You will need a prescription for any of these medicines. If you suspect a strep throat, see your mission doctor or a medical practitioner so you can be tested. The bacteria that cause strep throat can sometimes attack your heart or kidneys, so it is very important that you get the appropriate treatment if you have strep throat.

OTHER CAUSES OF SORE THROAT

Sometimes sore throats can be caused by fungal infections. This condition is called "thrush". The mouth and throat area are covered in a white, cheese-like pus that can be easily scraped off, leaving a red area. Individuals with these symptoms should be checked by a healthcare practitioner for appropriate diagnosis and treatment.

WHEN A SORE THROAT IS AN EMERGENCY

If someone with a sore throat has trouble breathing or feels that his or her throat is swelling shut, this individual may have a more serious problem and needs emergent medical attention. In addition, a person with a sore throat who has trouble swallowing, is drooling, or is choking should be checked by a healthcare practitioner as soon as possible.

SPRAINS AND STRAINS

The treatment for sprains and strains described in this section will be pertinent to most major joints. However, the images that accompany the text will be of the ankle, as the majority of sprains and strains occur at the ankle.

A sprain is an injury of ligaments caused by being stretched beyond their normal capacity. The ligaments may actually tear. Stretching a muscle beyond its normal capacity is referred to as a strain.

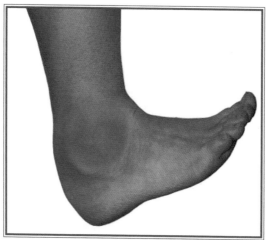

The typical signs and symptoms associated with a sprain or strain include:

- Inflammation
- Localized pain
- Swelling/discoloration

- Loss of normal limb function
- Decrease of joint flexibility

Sprains are graded in three degrees:

- A first degree sprain is only a minor tear or stretch of a ligament followed by minor pain.
- A second degree sprain is a tear of a ligament, which is usually followed by moderate pain, swelling, and/or discoloration. The joint may feel unstable.
- A third degree sprain is a complete rupture of the ligament and is accompanied by severe swelling and pain. The joint will likely feel unstable.

Some sprains can be severe enough to break the surrounding bones (4th or 5th degree). Even though these types of sprains can occur, they are less likely.

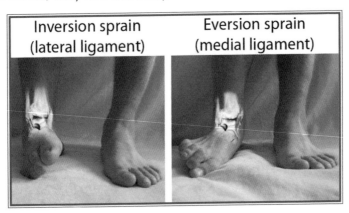

Inversion sprain (lateral ligament)   Eversion sprain (medial ligament)

TREATMENT

R.I.C.E

For all grades of ankle sprain follow the R.I.C.E. principles as soon as possible:

- **R**est your ankle or joint – do not walk on it.

- **I**ce – this helps to keep the swelling down. Use ice on the injury 4-5 times a day for 15-20 minutes each time.
- **C**ompression bandages are needed to immobilize the sprain and to support the injury. Compress joints to their active position (ankles 90 degrees, hands straight, etc.) for best ligament recovery.
- **E**levate the injury to a height at or above the level of your heart as much as possible for 48 hours.

Taking 800 mg of ibuprofen up to 3 times a day will help manage the pain and can help with inflammation. If you have a history of stomach ulcers or a kidney condition, ask a doctor before using ibuprofen.

If the sprain is a 2nd or 3rd degree sprain, seek medical attention immediately.

STIFF NECK

DESCRIPTION

Many missionaries will experience a stiff neck sometime while on their mission. Neck pain may feel like a "kink," stiffness, or severe pain. Pain may spread to the shoulders, upper back, or arms, or it may cause a headache. Neck movement may be limited, usually more on one side than the other. While the condition is typically nothing to worry about and does not require medical care, it can be, quite literally, a pain in the neck.

Neck pain is often caused by a strain or spasm of the neck muscles or inflammation of the neck joints. Examples of common activities that may cause this type of minor injury include:

- Holding the head in a forward, odd position while tracting, riding a bike (see Appendix D: Bike Setup), or even while reading.
- Sleeping on a pillow that is too high, too flat, or doesn't support your head.
- Sleeping on your stomach with your neck twisted or bent.
- Tension from stress may make the muscles on the back of the head and across the back of the shoulder feel tight.

TREATMENT

Luckily, there are many ways to soothe a stiff neck and speed up recovery. If a neck strain is suffered suddenly from an activity, such as basketball, apply only ice to the area of discomfort within the first 48 hours to help to decrease local inflammation and pain. Ice should be kept on for a maximum of 20 minutes and can be applied 3-4 times a day. A plastic bag with ice or a frozen bag of vegetables can be used.

If the neck pain comes on slowly over days, or if it's been more than 48 hours after a sudden injury, it is okay to use heat or ice as a first line of treatment. Relaxing the muscles with a hot shower or massage can help relieve a stiff neck as well. A hot water bottle or hot compress, made by soaking a towel in hot water, can also be applied to a stiff neck to aid in relaxation.

Gentle stretches and resistance exercises can help. Letting the weight off your head, allowing it to passively stretch in all directions, can help to loosen tight muscles and tendons. For example, if you have pain or tightness in the left side of your neck, you can let the head slowly fall to the right, giving a stretch to the left neck muscles.

Over-the-counter pain medications, such as aspirin, acetaminophen (Tylenol) / paracetamol, or ibuprofen (Advil), can be useful. Ibuprofen is preferred initially because it has anti-inflammatory properties.

If the neck pain/stiffness is accompanied by fevers, chills, severe headaches, sensitivity to light, nausea, vomiting, rash, and/or drowsiness, seek medical attention.

PREVENTION

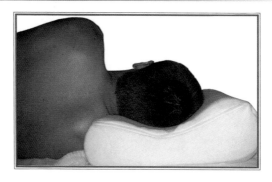

Stress, poor posture, bike riding and sleeping in the wrong position are all common causes of a stiff neck. Position your work, such as the books you are studying, at a level that allows you to hold your head in a normal, neutral position. Avoid activities that compress your neck, such as holding a phone between your head and shoulder. One thing you can try is to sleep with your neck straight, as shown in the picture. You can use a special pillow or use towels or sheets to align your neck in this manner.

SWINE FLU
(HINI Influenza)

See the chapter on influenza. Swine flu is just the name for a particular type of influenza virus (named for a similar flu virus that pigs can contract). Like other flu viruses, swine flu is very contagious and can spread rapidly from human to human. Symptoms of swine flu are similar to the symptoms of regular human flu described in the chapter on influenza. People with swine flu may also have additional symptoms of diarrhea or other atypical flu symptoms.

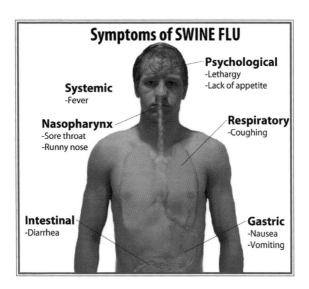

Whereas the annual season flu viruses are usually most severe in the very young and the very old, swine flu can cause severe disease in otherwise healthy young adults. If you suspect that you have the swine flu, contact the mission doctor.

TICKS

DESCRIPTION

Ticks are extremely small, hard-shelled insects that feed on the blood of animals and humans. They are found in areas with dense vegetation or they can transfer to humans from other mammals such as mice, dogs, and cats.

TICK-BORNE ILLNESSES

Ticks may transmit serious illnesses like Lyme disease, Tularemia, Rocky Mountain Spotted Fever, Babesiosis, Tick-borne Encephalitis, and Bartonella. If untreated, these diseases cause acute or chronic infections that can lead to long-term disability and even death.

Currently, 63 countries are considered endemic or potentially endemic for Lyme disease. The CDC estimates that 300,000 people are infected with Lyme disease every year in just the United States.

TREATMENT

Tick diseases usually require rapid treatment to avoid possible severe illness. Notify your mission president's wife and see a tick-borne disease doctor immediately if you have a suspected or known tick bite and exhibit any of the following signs or symptoms:

- Rash of any size or shape
- Fever/chills/vomiting/flu-like symptoms
- Severe body aches and pains

- Headaches
- Gastrointestinal symptoms
- New fatigue

TICK REMOVAL

Use your fingers or fine-tipped tweezers to grasp the tick as close to the skin's surface as possible and pull upward with a steady, even pressure. Do not twist or yank the tick as this could cause the mouth parts to break off and remain in the skin. After removing the tick, thoroughly clean the bite area and your hands with rubbing alcohol or soap and water. Do not use petroleum jelly, fingernail polish, rubbing alcohol, gasoline, matches, or a lighter to remove a tick.

Save the tick in a plastic bag with moistened paper or cotton ball and take it to your doctor. The tick may be sent to a special lab to test for infectious diseases.

PREVENTION

- Use insect repellents that contain >20% DEET and have your clothing soaked in Permethrin before your mission. When properly applied, Permethrin soaked clothing can deter ticks for many months. (See the appendix for more information.)
- Avoid wooded and bushy areas with high grass and leaf litter.
- Walk in the center of trails and avoid brushing against vegetation.
- Bathe or shower after coming indoors to wash off ticks that are not yet attached. Conduct a full-body check to look for ticks especially in the armpits, ears, belly button, groin area, behind the knees, around the waist, and in hair.
- Ticks can ride home on clothing and attach to a person later so carefully examine clothes, coats, and bags.

If possible, tumble clothes in a dryer on high heat for one hour to kill ticks.
- Be careful around any pets you encounter. Eliminate mice and rodents from your apartment.

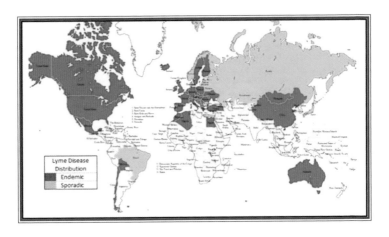

TOOTHACHE AND DENTAL PROBLEMS

TOOTHACHE

The common toothache is caused when the pulp (nerves and blood vessels in the tooth) becomes inflamed. Inflammation is the result of a cavity (decay) or an abscess (infection), and the sooner you can get treatment from a trained professional the better. However, you may be serving in an area where dental care is unavailable or scary at best. This chapter will give you some guidelines to treat yourself until you can see a trained dentist.

Sensitive teeth may cause discomfort or pain, but may not be the result of a cavity. If the tooth aches with hot or cold drinks or food, but returns to normal immediately after you have removed the stimulus, you probably just have sensitive teeth and not a cavity. Simply apply a 'sensitive formula' toothpaste (such as Sensodyne) to the teeth that are sensitive twice a day for 3-4 days. Place a pea size amount on your finger and rub it onto the sensitive tooth or teeth, and let it sit there for at least twenty minutes. If the sensitivity doesn't go away after 3-4 days or if the pain lingers on longer than 30 seconds when you drink cold drinks or hurts spontaneously, you should see a dentist.

If you are in an area that doesn't have a dentist and your tooth is hurting there are some things you can do to make the tooth more comfortable until you can see a dentist.

Ideas for pain management:

- Avoid foods that make the tooth ache; mostly hot, cold and sweets.
- Pain relief: Over-the-counter medicines such as aspirin, ibuprofen, and acetaminophen / paracetamol work well. Do not place aspirin directly on the tooth or gums, this will only damage (burn) the tissue and make matters worse.
- Place a temporary filling (see below)
- Keep the tooth clean

ABSCESS

Teeth that hurt when you chew or are tender to the touch may be developing an abscess. If your face, jaw line, or the tissue next to a tooth is swollen; you have an abscess. An abscess needs to be treated, usually by draining. Sometimes an abscess can drain spontaneously, but most often a dentist will need to do this. Pain medicines keep the tooth comfortable but they don't address the abscess. Antibiotics will be part of the treatment. Consult with a medical or dental professional before taking any antibiotics. If swelling is present and if there is a cavity in the tooth do not temporarily fill the tooth. If you fill the cavity, the abscess may not be able to drain and this can cause more pain.

LOST FILLING

If a filling comes out, it is usually because there is either decay under the filling or because the tooth or filling cracked.

- Wash your hands with soap and water
- Brush then rinse with warm water with salt in it or with mouthwash

- Fill the hole with a temporary filling material. You can use wax or even sugarless gum. Roll the material into a small ball and place it in the cavity and remove any excess. If a corner of the tooth or an entire side has broken away, fill the area in as best you can.
- Give pain medication as needed if you have pain.
- If unable to place a temporary filling, keep the tooth as clean as possible.

KNOCKED-OUT TOOTH

If a tooth is knocked out, quick action is needed to save the tooth. The longer the tooth is out of the mouth, the less the chance of survival for that tooth. If feasible, put the tooth back in its socket as soon as possible.

- Hold the top of the tooth.
- Rinse the tooth gently with warm clean water to remove any dirt.
- Do not scrub, disinfect, or let the root surface dry out.
- You may carefully pick off any stubborn debris.
- Gently place the tooth back into the socket. This may hurt.
- If the tooth is loose or mobile after re-implantation, stabilize the tooth by holding it gently in place with your finger and immediately find a dentist. If you don't have a dentist nearby, secure the tooth in position. You may have to be creative if you don't have a dentist nearby and use something like super glue or duct tape to hold it to an adjacent tooth.
- Do not chew anything hard on this tooth until you are able to get professional treatment.

If you don't replace the tooth immediately but can see a dentist within several hours, place the tooth in milk. If milk is not available, transport the tooth in your own saliva. Water is good for rinsing teeth, but not very good for transporting teeth.

TUBERCULOSIS (TB)

DESCRIPTION

Missionaries might encounter people with Tuberculosis (TB). This is an infection that is found in all parts of the world. TB is more common in parts of Central and South America, Africa, and Asia. Missionaries in these areas are likely to encounter people with this disease. TB is caused by an infection of slow-growing bacteria in organs that have a lot of blood and oxygen. That's why TB most often affects the lungs. But, TB can also spread to other parts of the body. If the lungs are infected with active TB, it is easy to spread the disease to others.

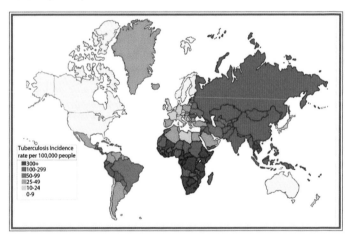

HOW IT IS SPREAD

TB in the lungs is contagious. It spreads when a person who has active TB breathes or coughs out air that has the TB bacteria in it, allowing others to breathe in the bacteria from the air.

A cough, sneeze, or laugh releases more bacteria than just quiet breathing. The bacteria can then remain airborne for hours. If TB is only in one part of the body, it does not spread easily to others.

TREATMENT

Doctors usually diagnose TB by doing a tuberculin skin test. During the skin test, a doctor or nurse will inject TB antigens under your skin. If you have TB bacteria in your body, you will get a red bump where the needle went into your skin within 2 days. If the skin test is positive or a cough is present, then a chest x-ray will also usually be done. Treatment is with specific antibiotics prescribed by a doctor.

PREVENTION

Be careful to keep your distance from people who are coughing. Be ready to say, "It looks like you aren't well today, so we'll come back when you're feeling better." Wash your hands often. Make sure to keep your immune system healthy by eating plenty of healthy foods, including fruits and vegetables, getting enough sleep, and exercising regularly. A great risk is sleeping in the same room with a companion who has active tuberculosis in their lungs. Signs and symptoms of active tuberculosis are fever, a cough that has gone on for more than 3 weeks, weight loss, sweating at nights when in bed, and a loss of appetite.

IMPORTANT: Tuberculosis can be dormant (silent) for a long time. It is very important that you be checked for tuberculosis by your doctor when you return home from your mission.

TYPHOID FEVER

BACKGROUND

If you have a high fever, diarrhea, headache and nausea, you might have typhoid fever. Be aware the diarrhea usually happens about one week after the other symptoms. This disease is found in all parts of the world including the United States, but it is more common in countries where sanitary conditions are poor. If you are serving in one of these countries, you might be infected with typhoid fever. This is a disease caused by bacteria. It is transmitted through eating food or drinking water that has been contaminated by the stools or urine of infected people.

SYMPTOMS

Symptoms usually develop 1–3 weeks after exposure and may be mild or severe. Typically, they include high fever, nausea, headache, constipation or diarrhea, and rose-colored spots on the chest. Typhoid fever can be treated with antibiotics. Cipro is the most common antibiotic used. This drug is used to treat a number of causes of diarrhea and fever. If you have these symptoms, speak with your mission doctor about using Cipro. In some areas, mostly Asia, doctors are using Azithromycin.

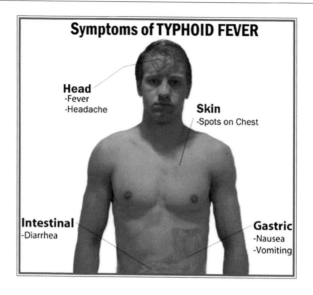

WORMS AND PARASITES

In many parts of the world, missionaries will be exposed to worms and parasites. Parasites are unable to produce food or energy for themselves. They are harmful to humans because they consume food, eat away body tissues, and create toxic waste that makes people sick. Worms and parasites are more common than you might think. Their presence causes a variety of chronic diseases and conditions such as chronic fatigue, weakness, low energy levels, skin rashes, pain, constipation, and frequent colds or influenza. There are two types of parasites: large and small.

Large Parasites

Large parasites, such as intestinal worms, are easily seen with the naked eye. These are roundworms, flukes, and tapeworms. Most worms grow outside of the body. However, some may lay their eggs on the intestinal walls. As the eggs hatch, the young larvae feed on the food in the intestinal tract. Intestinal worms sometimes dig through the digestive tract to get into the bloodstream, muscles, and other organs, where they cause even more havoc. These types of parasites often cause malnutrition and anemia (low blood levels) because they tend to rob the body of essential nutrients.

Small Parasites

Small parasites are so tiny that they can only be seen with a microscope. These tiny parasites are even more dangerous to the body than the large ones. Although they usually stay in the intestines, small parasites can migrate virtually anywhere in the body: into the bloodstream, muscles, and even vital organs such as the brain, the lungs, or the liver, where they do substantial damage.

Because parasites are everywhere, it is easy to become infected. Missionaries can become infected through:

- Insect bites
- Walking barefoot
- Eating raw or undercooked pork, beef or fish
- Eating contaminated raw fruits and vegetables
- Eating foods prepared by infected handlers
- Drinking contaminated water

There are more than 100 types of human parasites. The following describe some of the most common species in America.

Insects

In the United States, because of high sanitary standards and a temperate climate, parasitic insects do not flourish. Common bugs such as ticks, mites, fleas, lice, and bedbugs may cause intense itching in affected areas. They are a nuisance but not a major health risk. One exception is the deer tick, which is associated with Lyme disease. Other parasites, spread by mosquitoes, cause more serious diseases like western and eastern equine encephalitis, malaria, Dengue fever, and yellow fever.

Intestinal Parasites

Some of the most common intestinal parasites include:

- *Pinworms*- This is the most common parasitic infection in the United States. The worm resides in the colon, yet it lays eggs outside the body, usually near the anus, a process that causes severe itching. The disease can be transmitted from one individual to another through dirty hands and clothing.

- *Tapeworms*- The two most common tapeworms are pork tapeworm and beef tapeworm. These are caused by eating uncooked meat. Adult tapeworms may become quite big, some as long as 20 feet (6.1 m). Pork tapeworm is the more harmful. It often causes anemia and weight loss.
- *Protozoa*- (one-celled organisms) such as *Giardia lamblia, Entamoeba histolytica,* or *Cryptosporidium* are some of the most common and infectious parasites in the world. They can be transmitted through contaminated food and water. They can also be spread from one person to another. Cramps, watery diarrhea, abdominal pain, and serious weight loss are common symptoms of Giardia infection.

Diagnosis

Parasitic infections are difficult to diagnose because many patients exhibit only vague symptoms or no symptoms at all. The following symptoms, however, may indicate parasitic infections:

- Sudden changes in bowel patterns (e.g. constipation that changes to soft and watery stool).
- Constant rumbling and gurgling in the stomach area unrelated to hunger or eating.
- Heartburn or chest pain.
- Itching around the nose, ears, and anus, especially at night.
- Losing weight with constant hunger.

There are tests that doctors may perform that will diagnosis a worm or parasite infection.

TREATMENT AND PREVENTION

In missions where worms and parasites are a problem, the Church will provide medicines to help treat and prevent infections. Make sure you take the medicines that you are given. If symptoms worsen between taking doses of the medication, see the mission doctor and you might receive additional therapy.

The following guidelines will help you avoid worm and parasite infections:

- Make sure meat is cooked well before eating.
- Avoid drinking untreated water.
- Avoid being bitten by mosquitoes, ticks, and other insects.
- Eat a well-balanced diet with lots of fiber, vegetables, fruits, whole grains, nuts, and seeds. Good nutrition improves immune function and protects the body against parasitic invasion.

If you think that you have a worm or parasite infection, contact the mission doctor.

WOUNDS

Missionaries are likely to cut or injure their skin while serving a mission. This chapter will give some guidelines on how to treat skin injuries. Of course, the best treatment is to seek professional medical attention. But some wounds are small and you can treat them on your own. If you want to treat a wound on your own, or if it is too far to travel to a doctor, there are some steps you should take.

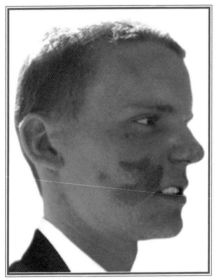

TREATMENT

The type of treatment necessary for each type of wound has the same basic principles:

Stop the Bleeding

The first task to perform is to stop the bleeding. Applying pressure to the wound is the best way to do this. For small wounds, you can use a simple bandage. For bigger wounds, you will need to press on the wound with your hand. Using the cleanest materials available, apply pressure to the source of the bleeding. Larger wounds may require direct pressure for several minutes. Scalp wounds may require pressure for a longer period of time.

If you can't stop the bleeding, you will need to seek medical attention quickly.

Prevent Infection

Infections can hinder the healing process and can also lead to life-threatening complications if not prevented. It is important to clean the wound thoroughly to avoid infection in the first place. This is usually done by irrigating the wound with water.

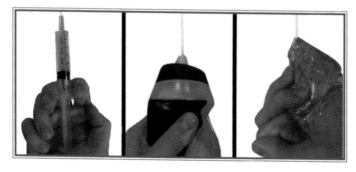

- Irrigate the wound with a forceful stream of clean water. One way to do this is to place the wound under a water tap. If you aren't near a tap, you can fill a plastic bag with water and cut a small hole in the side of it to create a stream of water.
- Gently pull apart the wound edges while you are irrigating to effectively remove all foreign matter and debris.

- It is important to note that irrigation may reinitiate bleeding. This is normal, but the bleeding must be stopped again.
- Abrasions that are very dirty may require vigorous scrubbing in order to remove dirt and other foreign material. Although scrubbing is painful, it is very important.

Protect the Wound

Bandaging a wound is very important to help preserve function and to minimize the scar that results from the wound. Sometimes a wound is a laceration (or ragged cut). The edges of the laceration will need to be brought together in some way. There are several effective ways to do this:

- Suturing (must be done by someone trained).
- Steri-strips, tape, or band-aids – bring the wound edges together and apply the steri-strip, band-aid, or tape across the wound.

Cover and Change the Dressing

Apply an antibiotic ointment to the wound and cover it up. All wounds should be covered with an ointment to keep them moist. Dressings should be changed daily or twice daily.

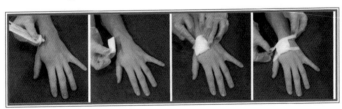

Immobilize the Wound

If the injury is on a flexible part of the body – an elbow or finger, for example – immobilize the joint with a splint to prevent reopening the wound.

TWO SPECIALIZED WOUNDS YOU SHOULD KNOW ABOUT

Puncture Wounds

If you step on a nail or something sticks into your skin, make sure you have had your tetanus shots. You should have been given a tetanus shot before you left on your mission.

- The area around the puncture site should be thoroughly scrubbed.
- Puncture wounds should be monitored more closely than simple lacerations, as they are at higher risk for infection.
- If the wound is not healing, or if you develop a fever, fast heart rate, or otherwise feel sick, you should see a doctor.

Deep Lacerations

- Managing deep lacerations on your legs or arms requires careful judgment because of the potential involvement of structures underneath the skin, such as tendons and nerves.

- Deep lacerations require that you seek medical help.

APPENDIX

APPENDIX A: PERMETHRIN

Missionaries in various parts of the world may find themselves sleeping on mattresses with fleas or other bugs such as scabies. Fleas and other insects that bite humans are everywhere. Often, these bites are only irritating, but at times the insect can spread disease. While most of the problems occur in certain parts of the world, bites can occur anywhere.

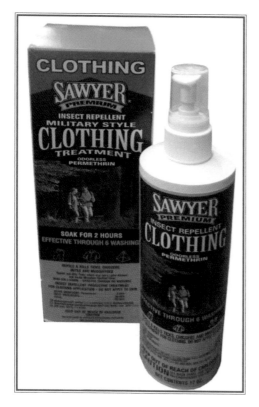

Permethrin was developed from a natural compound named pyrethrin, originally found in a flower. Permethrin is an odorless insecticide that can be sprayed on clothing and bedding. As a cream, it can also be applied to the skin. Permethrin prevents and treats insect-born infestations such as head lice and scabies. It can also be used to kill ticks and mosquitos.

Bed fleas are a huge problem in some missions. Fleas live in the mattresses and will bite the missionary as he or she sleeps. The main symptom of lice or fleas is itching. Soaking bedding in permethrin prevents bugs from biting, and one application to your bedding can last upwards of 3 or more months.

Currently, commercial airlines will not ship permethrin in personal luggage when leaving the MTC in Provo, Utah. The Church complies with this and asks that permethrin not be carried in luggage by missionaries as they leave that facility. If permethrin is not sold in travel or outdoor stores in your mission, ask the mission office or your parents to check to see if it may be shipped to your country via a secondary carrier such as DHL, FedEx, or UPS. Additionally, a missionary can soak clothing and bedding before he or she leaves for the mission field.

APPENDIX B: WATER DISINFECTION

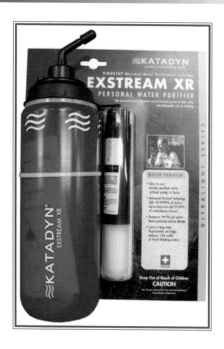

The Church has identified regions where the lack of clean water is a serious problem. In some areas, missionaries are provided with Seychelle water filtration bottles, bottled water, or equipment to treat water. If a program such as this has been established in your area, follow it closely. If you are in an area where you are required to disinfect water on your own, here are some guidelines to use as recommendations.

Drinking contaminated water can lead to diarrheal illness, parasite infection, dehydration, and chronic intestinal problems. The goal of water disinfection is to eliminate or reduce the number of infectious organisms to an acceptably low number so it does not cause you to be sick.

Waterborne organisms fall into four major categories:

- bacteria
- viruses
- protozoa (small one-celled organisms)
- worms

The likelihood of encountering any of these microorganisms depends on your location and on the exposure of the water source to contamination. Here are some methods of disinfecting water that you can use if needed.

1. Heat

Most organisms are readily destroyed by heat. Lower temperatures can be effective with longer contact times, and higher temperatures can be effective with shorter contact times.

The boiling point of water at sea level is 100°C (212°F). As soon as water has reached its boiling point temperature, it is sufficiently disinfected. In fact, the disinfection has generally occurred before the time the water boils. One important characteristic of boiling points is that they decrease in temperature with increasing elevation. The Center for Disease Control in the United States recommends boiling water for 3 minutes if one is located above 6,562 feet (2000 m).

2. Water Filters

Filters screen out bacteria, protozoa, and worms, but they are not very reliable for eliminating viruses.

Viruses tend to adhere to other particles or clump together, which helps remove some of them by filtration. Nevertheless, they are so small (less than 0.1 micron) that they cannot be eradicated by filters alone. Some filters are impregnated with iodine and bactericidal crystals in an attempt to destroy the viruses as they pass through the material. However, these additions are of questionable effectiveness.

Because filters work by trapping small particles in their pores, they can clog and become less effective over time. Operating a pump as it becomes clogged can force pathogens through it and contaminate the water. So, you need to be careful and know that filters should be used in addition to other disinfection methods.

3. Halogenation

Iodine and chlorine tablets can be very effective as disinfectants against viruses and bacteria. They are convenient in that missionaries can carry the tablets with them and treat water while away from their apartments. However, their effectiveness against worms and protozoa, as well as their eggs, varies greatly.

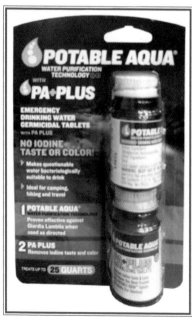

Disinfection depends on both iodine and chlorine concentration and contact time. Chlorine is more sensitive to these factors, and is thus less suitable for cold, contaminated water. In these conditions, both iodine and chlorine require increased contact time and/or concentration.

Though they can disinfect, another challenge with chlorine and iodine is the unpleasant taste they give to the water. This can be remedied in several ways, but must be done after disinfection. Adding a flavored drink mix or vitamin C can make the drink taste better. Activated charcoal can also be used to improve the taste of water after disinfection.

4. Ultraviolet Radiation (UVR)

UVR has gained popularity as a portable means of water disinfection. A UVR light source is inserted into water, which kills harmful organisms. However, UVR has some disadvantages. The units require batteries and can break easily. Despite these challenges, they are effective and are smaller than filters.

5. Chlorine Dioxide

Chlorine dioxide is another chemical compound used to disinfect water. It is safe and effective. It is available in both liquid and tablet form. It comes in a small bottle that is convenient for missionaries to carry with them.

HYGIENE

As a final note, washing hands and cleaning eating utensils is perhaps the most important thing a missionary can do to prevent intestinal illness. This means using warm, soapy water for cleaning. Eating and cooking utensils should be cleaned thoroughly after each use.

Alcohol-based hand sanitizers are very effective and sold in small containers that can easily be stored in a book bag or backpack. Remember that hand sanitizer should not be used as a replacement to thorough handwashing, nevertheless it is effective if your hands are not visibly dirty. Wash your hands often.

APPENDIX C:
FIRST AID KITS

As a missionary, you'll want to have a small first aid kit to help you take care of minor injuries and illnesses. It is not possible to create a medical kit that will cover every situation for every missionary. Some missionaries will find themselves in very remote areas where not only is access to medical care very limited, but access to a drug store is impossible. Here are some guidelines and suggestions to consider as you prepare a missionary first aid kit.

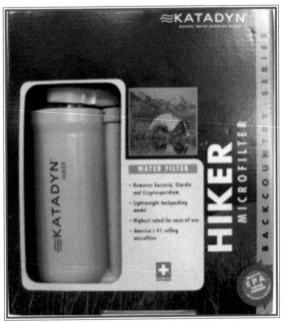

- You need to consider whether or not your mission has water contamination concerns. You may want to take

some water treatment options with you (see Appendix B for ideas). If youare in a high-risk area, it would be wise to take some water treatment chemicals that you can drop into water as needed.
- Consider the following for treatment of simple wounds:
  - Multiple sizes of bandages
  - Triple antibiotic ointment
  - Butterfly bandages
  - Gauze pads
  - Alcohol prep pads
  - Tape
  - Blistoban for blisters
  - Burn treatment gel

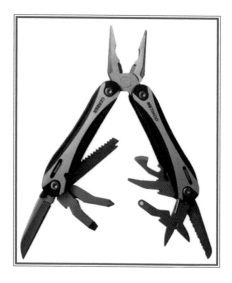

- Consider taking a multipurpose utility tool containing a knife, screwdrivers, scissors, pliers, tweezers, etc.
- Consider the following for dental care:
  - Dental filling material in case of a lost filling
  - Dental floss
  - An extra toothbrush
- Suggestions for medications to carry:
  - Prior to leaving, discuss a plan with your physician about any prescriptions you may need for chronic

conditions. Examples include medications for diabetes, heart conditions, severe allergies, psychiatric conditions, etc.

- Ibuprofen or acetimenophen for pain
- Antifungal skin cream
- Hydrocortisone 1% cream or ointment
- Afrin (oxymetazoline) nasal spray to stop nose bleeds and to help you breathe if you're infected with a virus
- Antihistamine for allergies
- Talk to your doctor about taking an antibiotic for a skin infection or some other kind of infection
- Eye drops
- Talk to your doctor about taking Cipro, an antibiotic used for treating diarrhea.
- Over-the-counter omeprazole or another antacid
- It is very important to avoid being bitten by insects. Here are some considerations of items that you might want to take:
  - Mosquito repellent
  - Permethrin is very useful but might have to be shipped to the area (see Appendix A: Permethrin)

APPENDIX D: BIKE SETUP

Many missionaries will use bicycles for a substantial part of their mission. Wearing a helmet, riding carefully, and being familiar with local traffic laws can help prevent many serious or even deadly accidents. In addition, proper bike setup and rider positioning can prevent muscle strains, a sore back, and many aches and pains. Though you can ride on a bicycle for a few hours without any discomfort, over time, an improper bike fit will almost guarantee things like burning feet, stabbing knee or back pain, sore hands, achy shoulders or a stiff neck.

Many bicycle shops will help you adjust your bike for free or for a small fee. It only takes a few minutes and is preferable if you have little or no experience adjusting a bicycle. If a bicycle shop is not available, or if you decide to adjust your bike on your own, here are a few tips. Some adjustments, such as seat height, will be made early on. Others, such as handlebar height, may require adjustment during the first few weeks on your bicycle. Note that these recommendations apply to a standard "mountain bike" style of bicycle.

1. Seat Height: While sitting on your bike seat, adjust the seat height such that when you have one leg extended straight, your heel is flush against the pedal. With this height, once you are pedaling with the balls of your feet, you will have the correct amount of knee flexion.

2. Seat Angle: Start with the seat parallel to the ground. If you experience discomfort, angle the seat up or down a few degrees until you are comfortable.

3. Handlebar Height: Comfort is the key. If your lower back, neck, hands, and/or arms hurt, you're probably leaning too far forward. If all your weight is on the seat and every bump hurts, you're sitting too upright. The handlebar height should be equal to the seat height, and no more than 3 - 4 inches lower than the seat height.

4. "Reach" (Seat to Handlebar Distance): Comfort is the deciding factor. Ideally, you'll be able to comfortably reach the handlebar without locking your elbows, without straining your back and/or neck, and without having to shift forward or back on the seat. Sit, and see how it feels. A good starting point is to be comfortable on the seat with your nose directly over the handlebars. Changing the reach requires installing a longer or shorter stem – the piece that holds the handlebars to the bike.

See chart for symptoms, potential causes, and solutions

Symptom	Potential Causes	Solution
Lower back pain	Stem too low or too long—must strain back to reach bars; seat may be too high, causing rocking when pedaling	Try raising the stem/handlebars; try installing a shorter stem; or check and adjust seat height
Constantly shifting forward on the seat	Stem may be too long, causing you to pull yourself forward as you ride; seat nose may be tipped down too much; seat may be too far back on its rails	Install a shorter stem; level saddle; move seat forward on rails

Constantly shifting back on the seat	Stem may be too short so you feel cramped and push yourself back; seat nose may be tipped up; seat may be too far forward on its rails	Install a longer stem; level the seat and center it on the rails; move your seat back
Neck pain	Stem too low, causing you to crane neck to see	Raise the stem/bars
Hands hurt	Stem too low, too much weight on hands; seat may be pointed down	Raise the stem/bars; level the seat
Front of knee hurts	Seat too low and/or tilted too far forward, straining knees	Raise the seat; may need to move seat further back as well
Back of knee hurts	Seat too high, over-extending leg	Lower the seat
Rear or crotch numbness or pain	Too much weight on the seat; may need to slide back a little on the seat	Lower handlebar position; check seat height as it may be too high; try sitting such that you feel the weight on the two lower bones of your pelvis rather than on the front or center of your crotch
Achilles tendon (back of foot) hurts	Pedaling too much on your toes	Keep the balls of your feet over the pedals when you're pedaling

INDEX

34295103R00084

Made in the USA
Lexington, KY
31 July 2014